THE COMPLETE GUIDE TO PEPTIDES FOR WOMEN

TABLE OF CONTENTS

TOOLS

Peptides by Purpose: A Summary
Peptide Tracker
Weekly Reflection
Weekly Habits Tracker
Weight Loss Tracker
Workout Journal
Food Journal
Wellness Tracker

INTRODUCTION

Why Peptides? Why Now?

Aging used to feel like a slow surrender. Fine lines. Sagging skin. Energy crashes that sneak up without warning. Weight gain that clings to your body no matter how many salads you eat or steps you count. For women, especially after 35 or 40, this shift often feels not just physical, but deeply personal. You wake up one day and no longer recognize the face in the mirror. The confidence you once wore like perfume starts to fade.

But what if aging didn't have to feel like decline? What if science has already handed us the tools to look better, feel sharper, and reclaim the vibrancy that once came effortlessly?

Enter: peptides.

Peptides are not magic pills. They are not another quick-fix trend flooding your feed with empty promises. They are short chains of amino acids—small but mighty molecules that your body naturally uses to send messages and spark regeneration.

As we age, ***our natural peptide production declines***, leading to slower repair, less collagen, more fat storage, and lower energy.

But the good news?

With targeted peptide therapy, you can help your body remember how to act young again.

So why now? ***The science is finally catching up with our desires.*** Just a decade ago, peptides were hidden behind clinical trials, elite clinics, and confusing medical jargon. Today, they are becoming more accessible to women everywhere through safe telehealth platforms, evidence-based protocols, and a growing movement of biohackers who are rewriting the rules of aging.

More importantly, we are entering a moment where women are no longer content with one-size-fits-all wellness. ***We know that female physiology is different.*** Our hormones, metabolism, and skin age differently from men's. We face unique challenges, all of which peptides can help support.

You might already be taking collagen powders, adaptogens, or hormone-balancing supplements. Maybe you've tried laser facials or lip fillers.

But peptides work on a deeper, more foundational level. ***They activate your body's repair systems from within.***

Some peptides stimulate growth hormone for fat loss and recovery. Others rebuild collagen to smooth wrinkles. Some calm inflammation, promote deeper sleep, or even reignite your sex drive.

This book is here to guide you through all of it, without the fluff. It is built for women who want real answers and smart, personalized strategies. Whether you are bio-curious, health-savvy, or just tired of feeling tired, you are not alone.

We'll explore the most effective peptides for female beauty, energy, and fat loss. ***We'll break down the science in plain language.*** You'll find step-by-step guidance for stacking, cycling, and even choosing the right protocols for your goals.

You are not broken. You are not done.

And you are not too late.

The time to feel radiant, strong, and powerful again is now. Peptides are not about perfection. They are about potential—the potential for your body to heal, glow, and thrive from the inside out.

Let's begin.

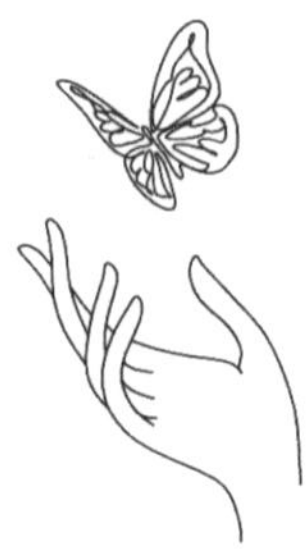

Breaking the Age Myth: A Biohacker's Manifesto

There is a myth we have been told since girlhood. It whispers in birthday cards that joke about getting older. It hides in creams that promise to "fight time." It lurks in the sighs we hear when another wrinkle appears or another strand of hair turns gray.

This myth says that beauty fades. That energy disappears. That aging is a steady descent, especially for women.

But what if that story was never written for you? What if it was based on outdated science, male-centered studies, and a cultural script designed to keep women quiet, compliant, and invisible past a certain age?

It is time to flip the narrative.

This is your biohacker's manifesto. And it begins with this belief: ***aging is not your enemy.*** It is not a process you are doomed to endure. It is a biological conversation—one you can actively shape, influence, and improve.

The modern woman is not content with declining slowly. She is not satisfied with surface-level solutions. She wants longevity with vitality, confidence without compromise, and beauty that reflects her strength, not her age. Biohacking gives you that power.

Biohacking is the art and science of optimizing your body using cutting-edge knowledge, tools, and strategies. It means understanding how your body works and then enhancing that system in smart, precise ways.

For men, biohacking often looks like testosterone and cold plunges. But your hormones cycle. Your needs shift. You don't just want to "perform better." You want to feel ***balanced, whole, and empowered***—in your skin, your energy, and your relationships.

Peptides are one of the most powerful tools in the female biohacker's toolkit. Why?

Peptides communicate directly with your body's repair systems. They remind your cells how to behave like they once did, when your skin was smooth, your body lean and your mind sharp.

They help reverse the signs of aging, not by masking them, but by repairing the systems behind them.

It is time to rethink what we've been told about aging.

Weight gain is not just about willpower.
It's often the result of hormonal shifts that change how your body stores fat.

Fatigue is not just in your mind.
It's linked to mitochondrial decline and chronic inflammation that slow down your energy systems.

Skin elasticity is not just a matter of luck.
It's directly tied to collagen production, which peptides like GHK-Cu can naturally stimulate.

This book is not a shallow guide to looking younger. It is a deeper invitation to ***feel stronger, sleep better, think clearer, and live bolder***. It challenges the lie that life peaks in your 20s. It celebrates the fact that with the right protocols, you can look and feel better at 45 than you did at 25.

This is the age of regenerative medicine, where we don't just treat symptoms, we heal systems. It is the age of female-centered wellness, where your body's rhythms are honored, not ignored. And it is the age of data-backed results, not guesswork.

You will not be asked to starve yourself. You will not be told to erase your natural features. Instead, ***you will learn to work with your biology.*** To activate your inner healer. To glow from within—not with trends or filters—but with ***cellular health, peptide precision, and confidence born from knowledge***.

This manifesto is not just about living longer. It is about living better, on your terms, in your power.

So let us end the myth. Let us stop
apologizing for wanting more.

More strength. More beauty.
More desire. More energy. More life.

Because ***you deserve to age boldly, brilliantly, and unapologetically.***

This is your moment. Biohack it.

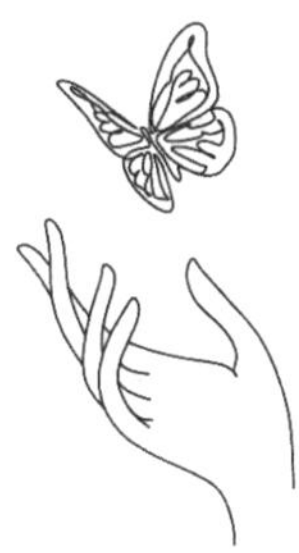

Part I: Foundations of Peptide Science

What Are Peptides?

In the world of advanced wellness, peptides have emerged as one of the most exciting and effective tools for optimizing health, reversing signs of aging, and enhancing overall vitality. But to truly unlock their power, you need to understand what peptides are, how they function in the body, and why they matter—especially for women.

Understanding Peptides

While proteins are long, complex chains made up of many amino acids, peptides are simpler—usually made of 2 to 50 amino acids. This is part of why they're so powerful and precise.

At their core, peptides are short chains of amino acids. Think of them as tiny messengers that tell your body what to do.

In biological terms, peptides act as signaling molecules. They bind to specific receptors on the surface of cells and trigger targeted actions—like stimulating collagen production, increasing fat metabolism, accelerating tissue repair, or boosting human growth hormone (HGH) release.

These natural chemical messengers are already found within your body, playing critical roles in regulating hormones, immunity, digestion, skin health, and neurological functions.

But as you age, your body produces fewer peptides, leading to slower recovery, duller skin, weight gain, fatigue, and other signs of aging.

Peptide therapy involves introducing bio-identical or synthetic peptides into the body to ***restore or enhance specific biological functions***. Unlike traditional pharmaceuticals that may have broad, systemic effects (and often side effects), ***peptides are targeted and specific. They do one job and do it well.***

Peptides vs. Proteins vs. Amino Acids

Let's break it down:

Molecule	Structure	Function	Size
Amino Acid	Single unit	Building blocks of proteins and peptides	Smallest
Peptide	2–50 amino acids	Signals biological actions (hormone release, healing, etc)	Medium
Protein	50+ amino acids, complex folding	Structural or functional (enzymes, transport, support)	Largest

This distinction is key. ***Amino acids are like letters. Peptides are short words. Proteins are full paragraphs.***

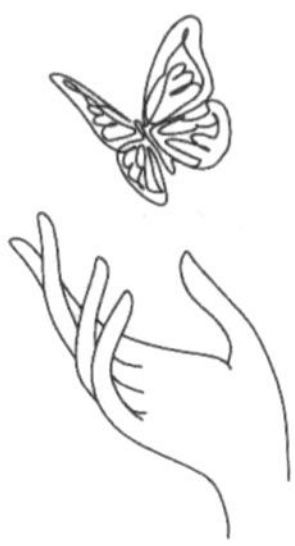

How Peptides Work in the Body

Once introduced (through injection, oral tablet, nasal spray, or topical application) peptides bind to receptors on cell surfaces.

Each peptide is designed to mimic or enhance the function of a natural peptide in your body.

Some examples:

GHK-Cu: Found naturally in plasma, this peptide binds with copper and stimulates collagen and elastin production, making it a superstar for skin rejuvenation.

BPC-157: The "body protection compound" promotes tissue repair and reduces inflammation, especially in the gut, joints, and muscles.

CJC-1295 + Ipamorelin: These peptides work together to stimulate growth hormone release, which helps burn fat, improve sleep, and restore muscle tone.

Semaglutide: Though technically a GLP-1 receptor agonist and not a classic peptide, it mimics the GLP-1 hormone to reduce appetite and regulate blood sugar, aiding in sustainable fat loss.

Peptides do not override your biology—they enhance and support it. This makes them uniquely suited for women looking to restore balance without aggressive pharmaceutical intervention.

Why Peptides Matter for Women

Female aging is hormonal, cellular, and multifactorial. Menopause and perimenopause shift estrogen, progesterone, and testosterone levels, leading to a cascade of effects: dry skin, weight gain, poor sleep, low libido, mood swings, brain fog, and more.

Peptides offer a ***customized toolkit*** for managing these shifts with precision:

Goal	**Best Peptides**	**Benefits**
Skin Tightening & Wrinkle Reduction	GHK-Cu, Matrixyl, SNAP-8	Boosts collagen, reduces lines, improves skin tone
Fat Loss & Metabolism	CJC-1295 + Ipamorelin, Semaglutide, Tirzepatide	Burns fat, controls hunger, promotes lean muscle
Libido & Hormonal Balance	PT-141, Kisspeptin-10, Oxytocin	Enhances sexual desire, improves mood, balances hormones
Healing & Recovery	BPC-157, TB-500	Repairs tissue, reduces inflammation, supports gut health
Cognitive Focus & Energy	Selank, Semax	Boosts dopamine, improves memory, stabilizes mood

These peptides do not just offer short-term fixes. They support **deeper regenerative processes**, helping your body to rebuild and perform better over time.

Delivery Methods and Bioavailability

How peptides are introduced into the body impacts their effectiveness. Here are the most common methods:

Subcutaneous Injection: The most effective and direct route. Delivered just under the skin using a small insulin syringe.

Topical Creams/Serums: Best for skin-related peptides like GHK-Cu or cosmetic formulations.

Nasal Sprays: Useful for brain-targeted peptides like Selank and Semax.

Oral Capsules: Some peptides can survive digestion and are formulated for oral absorption, though effectiveness varies.

Transdermal Patches: An emerging field for sustained peptide delivery through the skin.

The method you choose depends on your goals and the specific peptide being used. For example, fat-loss peptides often require daily or weekly injections, while beauty peptides might be used topically.

Is Peptide Therapy Safe?

Yes, when used responsibly and under medical guidance, peptide therapy is considered safe. Most peptides mimic naturally occurring substances in the body, which reduces the risk of rejection or serious side effects.

However, sourcing matters. You must use peptides from licensed compounding pharmacies or telehealth clinics that ensure purity and quality. Avoid online gray-market peptides that may be contaminated, underdosed, or mislabeled.

Side effects are rare but can include:

- Injection site irritation
- Mild fatigue or headaches (depending on the peptide)
- Water retention (especially with growth hormone secretagogues)

Proper cycling, dosage, and periodic breaks can reduce the chance of side effects and ensure long-term benefits.

Peptides are not hype. They are the next evolution in wellness science. Small enough to go unnoticed, but powerful enough to reset your systems, peptides offer women a new way to engage with their biology —intelligently, gently, and with real results.

In the chapters ahead, we'll explore each peptide in detail—how it works, what it does, and how it fits into your personal protocol.

But for now, just remember this: ***Peptides give you the opportunity to feel like yourself again—only stronger, clearer, and more radiant than ever before.***

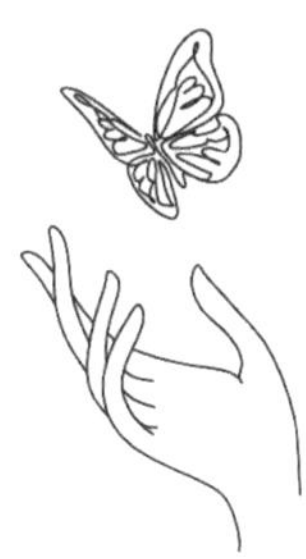

The Female Body and Peptides: A Perfect Match

Women's bodies are rhythmic, responsive, and intricately designed. From menstruation and pregnancy to perimenopause and beyond, hormonal shifts shape nearly every aspect of a woman's physical and emotional health. This ever-evolving biology is precisely why peptides are such a powerful tool for female wellness.

Peptides communicate with your body in a way that aligns beautifully with the needs of a woman. They can be selective, gentle, and specific—ideal qualities for supporting a body that thrives on balance rather than brute force.

Unlike many pharmaceutical drugs that override systems, peptides work with your natural pathways to restore what time, stress, and hormones may have disrupted.

Take collagen, for instance. As estrogen declines with age, so does collagen production, leading to thinner skin, fine lines, and loss of elasticity. Peptides like ***GHK-Cu*** step in and signal the skin to start rebuilding collagen and repairing damage—without introducing synthetic hormones.

This is precision beauty, from the inside out.

Or consider ***BPC-157***, which has become a favorite for women dealing with ***gut inflammation***, joint pain, or slow tissue healing. Whether from exercise, autoimmune flare-ups, or simply aging, this peptide encourages regeneration where your body needs it most—without the side effects of steroids or painkillers.

Women also experience unique challenges in ***body composition***. Menopause and perimenopause often trigger fat storage in the midsection, even when diet and exercise stay consistent. Growth hormone-releasing peptides like ***CJC-1295 and Ipamorelin*** help regulate metabolism, improve sleep quality, and promote lean muscle, giving women the tools to reshape their bodies at any age.

Sexual wellness is another area where peptides shine. With age, libido often declines, not because of disinterest but due to hormonal shifts, blood flow issues, and emotional exhaustion. Peptides like ***PT-141 and Kisspeptin-10*** help rekindle sexual desire, arousal, and pleasure—all without altering your baseline hormones.

And let's not forget the brain. From mood swings and brain fog to anxiety and poor sleep, women are more likely than men to experience neurologically driven symptoms throughout life. ***Cognitive peptides*** like ***Selank and Semax*** gently support mood regulation, stress resilience, and mental clarity.

In short, peptides are a woman's secret ally. They're smart, adaptable, and deeply aligned with the nuances of female physiology.

Your body is not broken. It's dynamic. And peptides are the language it understands.

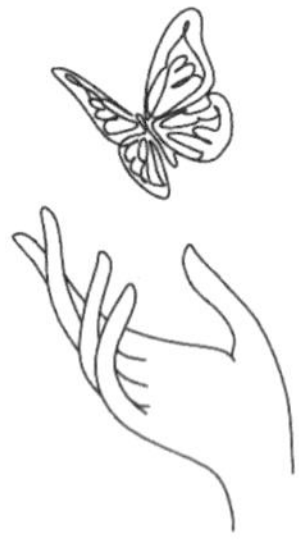

Hormones, Aging, and Cellular Repair: A Medicine Approach

Aging is often portrayed as a linear process—wrinkles appear, energy fades, metabolism slows, and hormone levels drop.

But through the lens of functional medicine, aging is far more dynamic. It's more than just about time passing, including ***how systems shift, interact, and compensate***. And when it comes to aging in women, the biggest players are hormones, inflammation, and cellular damage.

Your body runs on biochemical messengers. Estrogen, progesterone, testosterone, insulin, thyroid hormones, cortisol—they orchestrate everything from metabolism and mood to skin regeneration and fat storage.

When one of these messenger hormones falls out of balance, the rest must adapt. That's why women often feel "off" even when basic lab tests come back "normal."

Functional medicine views these symptoms not as isolated problems, but as clues from an interconnected system. ***It asks why your skin is thinning, why you're gaining weight, or why your libido disappeared,*** rather than masking it with a quick fix.

One of the most critical root causes? Cellular dysfunction.

As you age, your mitochondria—the tiny power plants inside each cell—start to falter. They produce less energy, leading to fatigue, slower metabolism, and even brain fog. Peptides like MOTS-c and SS-31 are being studied for their ability to rejuvenate mitochondrial function and improve cellular vitality.

Inflammation is another silent accelerator of aging. Chronic low-grade inflammation (often triggered by diet, stress, toxins, or leaky gut) can damage cells, disrupt hormones, and lead to weight gain, fatigue, and autoimmune flare-ups. Peptides like BPC-157 and Thymosin Alpha-1 have shown promise in reducing systemic inflammation.

And then there's ***collagen loss***. Starting in your 30s, your ability to produce collagen and elastin begins to drop, leading to sagging skin, joint pain, and poor wound healing. Peptides such as GHK-Cu and Epitalon support DNA repair and collagen synthesis, helping reverse this process in a way that feels natural and lasting.

Hormonal shifts during perimenopause and menopause can also disrupt sleep, mood, and metabolism. Functional medicine supports using lifestyle interventions, nutrient support, and peptides to ***restore balance without overriding your natural systems***. For example, Sermorelin encourages your body to increase its own growth hormone production, rather than replacing it entirely.

Functional medicine and peptides go hand in hand because they share a common philosophy: support the body's ability to heal itself, rather than imposing solutions that suppress symptoms.

This approach invites you to become an active participant in your wellness, not just a passive recipient of prescriptions. You track, adjust and listen to your body's responses. Over time, you create a protocol that's uniquely yours.

Aging does not have to mean decline. When you repair at the cellular level, rebalance your hormones, and reduce inflammation, you do not just look younger—you feel younger.

Functional medicine gives you the map. Peptides are the tools. And your body? It's ready to do the work.

Part II: Peptides for Beauty, Skin, and Hair

Reclaiming Your Skin's Youth

Aging skin tells a story. It speaks of time, environment, stress, and the body's natural hormonal shifts. ***Fine lines, wrinkles, sagging, and dryness are signals from deep within***, often pointing to one crucial issue: the gradual decline in collagen production. This is where GHK-Cu steps into the spotlight.

What is GHK-Cu?

GHK-Cu is a copper peptide. Discovered in human plasma, it is a naturally occurring molecule composed of amino acids bonded with copper.

What makes GHK-Cu remarkable is its ability to communicate directly with your cells, triggering them to begin regeneration and repair.

As we age, the natural levels of GHK-Cu in our body drop significantly. By age 60, the levels can decrease by more than 60 percent, which is why introducing GHK-Cu can be so effective.

And then there's ***collagen loss***. Starting in your 30s, your ability to produce collagen and elastin begins to drop, leading to sagging skin, joint pain, and poor wound healing. Peptides such as GHK-Cu and Epitalon support DNA repair and collagen synthesis, helping reverse this process in a way that feels natural and lasting.

Hormonal shifts during perimenopause and menopause can also disrupt sleep, mood, and metabolism. Functional medicine supports using lifestyle interventions, nutrient support, and peptides to ***restore balance without overriding your natural systems***. For example, Sermorelin encourages your body to increase its own growth hormone production, rather than replacing it entirely.

Functional medicine and peptides go hand in hand because they share a common philosophy: support the body's ability to heal itself, rather than imposing solutions that suppress symptoms.

Benefits of GHK-Cu for Skin Health

1. **Stimulates Collagen & Elastin Production**

   GHK-Cu reactivates genes that were once active in younger skin, prompting the synthesis of collagen and elastin. This leads to visibly firmer, smoother skin.

2. **Improves Skin Tightness and Texture**

   Regular application can reduce fine lines, tighten loose skin, and restore softness and evenness to skin tone.

3. **Reduces Photodamage and Pigmentation**

   GHK-Cu has been shown to repair DNA damage caused by UV rays, helping to fade sunspots and even out skin tone.

4. **Supports Wound Healing and Scar Reduction**

   This peptide is often used post-procedures or for chronic wounds, as it speeds up healing and reduces inflammation.

5. **Enhances Overall Skin Glow**

   Many users report a noticeable radiance and "plumped" appearance within weeks of use.

What Makes GHK-Cu Unique Among Skincare Peptides?

- It carries copper directly to cells, enhancing enzymatic function and energy production.
- It supports over 4,000 genes related to tissue remodeling.
- It not only protects but reverses visible signs of skin damage.
- It works for women of all skin types and ages, including postmenopausal skin.

What to Expect

Most users notice subtle improvements in tone and hydration within 2 to 3 weeks. Deeper results—such as firmer skin, reduced lines, and more elasticity—typically take 8 to 12 weeks of consistent use.

These results are cumulative, not temporary, which means your skin continues to improve over time.

GHK-Cu is not just a cosmetic enhancer. It is a cellular communicator that invites your skin to regenerate from within. In a world filled with flashy serums and surface-level treatments, this peptide works at the root, by awakening your skin's memory of youth.

You do not have to accept dullness, sagging, or premature aging as inevitable. With the right tools, including GHK-Cu, you can support your skin's natural intelligence and reclaim the glow, strength, and softness that reflects your inner vitality. This is not about chasing youth. It is about supporting beauty that lasts, because it is built on real healing and real repair, not illusion.

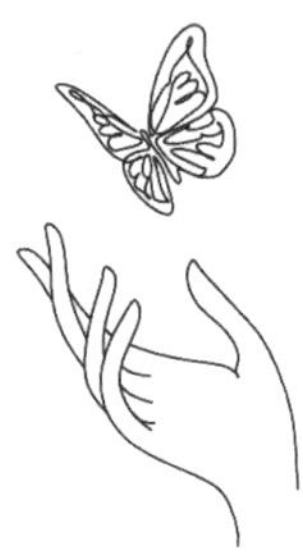

The Non-Surgical Facelift

As we age, the skin begins to lose its structure. Collagen depletes, elastin weakens, and moisture retention declines. This gradual breakdown results in visible sagging, fine lines, and deep wrinkles—especially around the jawline, cheeks, and eyes.

While surgical facelifts once seemed like the only path to rejuvenation, science has now introduced safer, less invasive options. Among the most promising tools? Peptides.

Peptides offer a ***non-surgical path to tighter, firmer, more youthful-looking skin*** by addressing the biological causes of aging—at the cellular level. Rather than stretching or filling the skin, they stimulate your body to restore its own structure.

How Peptides Tighten and Rejuvenate Skin

Peptides like GHK-Cu, Matrixyl (palmitoyl pentapeptide), Argireline, and SNAP-8 work by mimicking or enhancing natural processes. These peptides signal ***fibroblasts*** (the skin's repair cells) to increase their activity, resulting in tighter skin and reduced creases over time.

- *GHK-Cu promotes collagen, elastin, and glycosaminoglycan synthesis while repairing damaged DNA and calming inflammation.*
- *Matrixyl is known to trigger the production of collagen and hyaluronic acid, making it ideal for deep wrinkle repair.*
- *Argireline and SNAP-8 are sometimes referred to as "Botox in a bottle" because they reduce the depth of wrinkles by relaxing facial tension.*

Best Practices for a Non-Surgical Facelift Routine

To maximize the effects of peptide therapy:

- ***Use a multi-peptide serum daily,*** especially formulations that combine GHK-Cu with Matrixyl or SNAP-8.
- ***Pair with microneedling or dermarolling*** (1–2 times per week) to boost peptide absorption and trigger deeper skin regeneration.
- ***Support from within*** by ensuring adequate protein intake, sleep, and hydration, all of which improve skin elasticity.
- ***Avoid harsh treatments*** that inflame or over-exfoliate the skin, as they can counteract the benefits of peptides.

And then there's ***collagen loss***. Starting in your 30s, your ability to produce collagen and elastin begins to drop, leading to sagging skin, joint pain, and poor wound healing. Peptides such as GHK-Cu and Epitalon support DNA repair and collagen synthesis, helping reverse this process in a way that feels natural and lasting.

Hormonal shifts during perimenopause and menopause can also disrupt sleep, mood, and metabolism. Functional medicine supports using lifestyle interventions, nutrient support, and peptides to ***restore balance without overriding your natural systems***. For example, Sermorelin encourages your body to increase its own growth hormone production, rather than replacing it entirely.

Functional medicine and peptides go hand in hand because they share a common philosophy: support the body's ability to heal itself, rather than imposing solutions that suppress symptoms.

Realistic Expectations

Peptides do not offer a dramatic overnight transformation. What they offer is more natural, graceful progress. Within 4 to 8 weeks, you may begin to notice:

- A firmer feel to the skin
- Fewer visible fine lines
- A more lifted appearance around the eyes or jaw
- Improved skin tone and texture

By 12 to 16 weeks, these changes often become more pronounced and lasting. Your face may not look ***surgically altered***—but it will look rested, vibrant, and authentically refreshed.

In a culture obsessed with extremes, peptides offer a smarter, subtler way to reclaim youthful skin—without going under the knife.

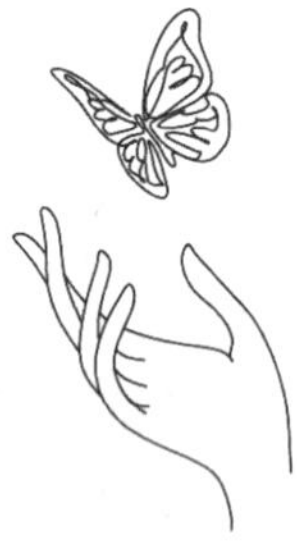

Hair Regrowth for Women

Hair loss in women can feel deeply personal. Whether it's a widening part, thinning at the crown, or excessive shedding, it often comes with emotional weight.

Unlike men, female hair loss is typically more diffuse and can be harder to treat. Hormonal fluctuations, stress, aging, nutrient deficiencies, and inflammation all play a role.

Thankfully, peptides offer a modern, science-backed solution. Peptides support hair growth not by masking symptoms, but by reactivating dormant hair follicles, improving blood flow, and repairing the scalp environment. For women seeking a non-hormonal and non-invasive treatment, these molecules are game-changers.

How Peptides Promote Hair Regrowth

Hair growth occurs in cycles: growth (anagen), transition (catagen), rest (telogen), and shedding (exogen).

Aging and hormonal imbalances shorten the growth phase and extend the resting phase. Peptides help by reversing this shift and bringing follicles back to life.

The most effective hair-regenerating peptides include:

- **GHK-Cu**: Known for increasing blood flow to the scalp, reducing inflammation, and stimulating the production of proteins essential for follicle health.
- **PTD-DBM and Valproic Acid (VPA)**: Shown in studies to stimulate the Wnt signaling pathway, which is crucial for hair regeneration.
- **Thymosin Beta-4 (TB-500)**: Enhances angiogenesis (new blood vessel formation) and supports cellular repair in the scalp.
- **BPC-157**: Useful when hair loss is related to autoimmune conditions or chronic inflammation.

These peptides do not merely thicken hair—they improve scalp health, stimulate cellular turnover, and extend the anagen phase for longer, healthier strands.

Delivery Methods and What Works Best

Topical applications are ideal for hair regrowth, especially serums or foams that contain GHK-Cu and other peptides in liposomal form for deeper penetration. For more advanced therapy, microneedling or dermarolling the scalp 1–2 times weekly improves absorption and encourages follicular stimulation.

Injectable mesotherapy, where small doses of peptides are injected into the scalp using micro-needles, is also gaining popularity in clinical settings. This method is more targeted and can yield faster results under professional supervision.

What to Expect and How Long It Takes

Hair regrowth is a slow and steady process. Most women begin to notice a reduction in shedding within 4–6 weeks. Visible regrowth usually takes 3 to 6 months, depending on the cause and severity of the hair loss. With continued use, strands become thicker, fuller, and healthier.

Support Your Hair from Within

Peptides work best when combined with a healthy scalp and lifestyle. Supporting nutrients include biotin, vitamin D, iron, and omega-3s. Reduce inflammation, manage stress, and avoid harsh chemical treatments for optimal results.

In summary, peptide therapy opens the door to real, visible renewal for women ready to take control of hair loss naturally.

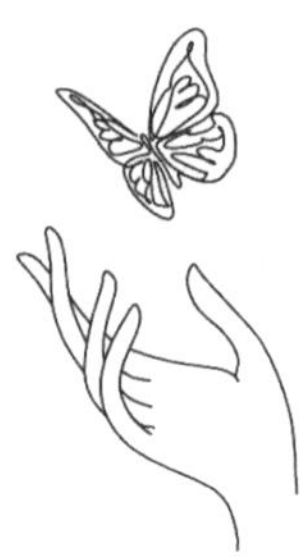

Unlocking the Youthful Glow

That healthy, luminous glow often associated with youth isn't magic but biology. Skin that radiates softness and vibrancy is deeply hydrated, collagen-rich, and well-nourished at the cellular level. Over time, stress, sun damage, poor sleep, and hormone decline dull that glow. Peptides, both topical and injectable, can restore it.

What Is a "Youthful Glow"?

A glowing complexion reflects light evenly across the skin. It is ***smooth, elastic, and free of fine lines, dry patches, and inflammation.*** This glow depends on three things:

1. Collagen and elastin content
2. Cellular hydration and renewal
3. Healthy circulation and barrier function

Peptides can influence all three.

Topical Peptide Protocols

The most accessible form of peptide therapy comes through serums and creams. Look for formulations containing:

- **GHK-Cu**: Boosts collagen, evens tone, and increases skin firmness.
- **Matrixyl (palmitoyl pentapeptide)**: Promotes smoother, wrinkle-free texture.
- **Argireline:** Relaxes facial muscles, softening expression lines.
- **Snap-8**: Reduces depth of fine lines and crow's feet.

Apply peptides to clean skin once or twice daily. For best results, pair with a hyaluronic acid serum to enhance absorption and lock in moisture. Always follow with sunscreen, as peptides make skin more photosensitive during repair cycles.

Weekly *microneedling* can increase penetration, helping peptides reach deeper layers of the dermis where regeneration occurs. This method is especially effective when targeting dullness, acne scars, and hyperpigmentation.

Delivery Methods and What Works Best

Topical applications are ideal for hair regrowth, especially serums or foams that contain GHK-Cu and other peptides in liposomal form for deeper penetration. For more advanced therapy, microneedling or dermarolling the scalp 1–2 times weekly improves absorption and encourages follicular stimulation.

Injectable mesotherapy, where small doses of peptides are injected into the scalp using micro-needles, is also gaining popularity in clinical settings. This method is more targeted and can yield faster results under professional supervision.

What to Expect and How Long It Takes

Hair regrowth is a slow and steady process. Most women begin to notice a reduction in shedding within 4–6 weeks. Visible regrowth usually takes 3 to 6 months, depending on the cause and severity of the hair loss. With continued use, strands become thicker, fuller, and healthier.

Morning

- Cleanser
- GHK-Cu serum + hyaluronic acid
- Vitamin C antioxidant serum
- Moisturizer + SPF

Evening

- Cleanser
- Matrixyl or SNAP-8 cream
- Retinol (alternate nights)
- Peptide sleeping mask

Weekly

- Microneedling (0.5 mm) with peptide serum application
- Hydrating sheet mask

Glow is not just a surface phenomenon but the result of cellular activity working in harmony. Peptides offer a targeted, non-disruptive way to activate this harmony. Whether through a luxurious topical serum or a professional injectable protocol, peptides support real renewal beneath the skin, allowing your radiance to shine through.

Forget filters. With peptides, the glow is real.

And it is yours to reclaim.

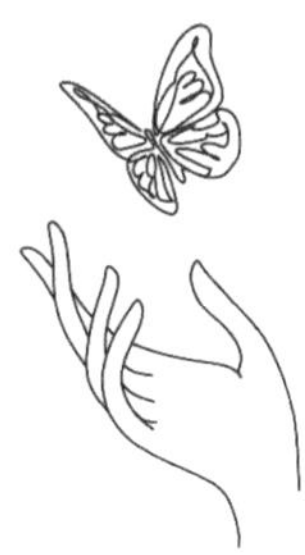

Part III: Peptides for Fat Loss and Body Composition

Breaking Through Belly Fat

Stubborn belly fat is one of the most frustrating parts of aging for women. It resists diet, ignores exercise, and often seems to appear overnight. But here's the truth: it is not just a matter of willpower or calories. Belly fat is strongly influenced by **hormonal shifts, stress response, insulin resistance, and inflammation**, all of which change drastically with age.

Peptides offer a unique solution by going under the surface to correct the biological patterns driving fat accumulation. Unlike stimulant-based fat burners, peptides work with your body's chemistry to restore balance, increase metabolism, and unlock stored fat for energy.

Why Belly Fat Happens—Especially to Women

In perimenopause and menopause, estrogen drops, and cortisol tends to rise. This hormonal imbalance signals your body to store fat, especially in the midsection. At the same time, your growth hormone levels decline, leading to slower metabolism and reduced lean muscle.

This triple threat—low estrogen, high cortisol, and reduced HGH—creates the perfect storm for fat gain. Peptides help by reigniting the metabolic fire that time and hormones try to extinguish.

Where Peptides Excel

- Midsection slimming without muscle loss
- Sustainable metabolic improvements
- Deeper sleep and better recovery, which support weight loss
- Hormonal harmony that makes weight loss easier and more natural

Top Fat-Burning Peptides for Women

- **CJC-1295 + Ipamorelin**: These two are often used together to stimulate your own growth hormone release. This leads to improved fat oxidation, better sleep, and muscle preservation. Women often report smoother body composition, even without drastic diet changes.

- Tesamorelin: Known for reducing visceral (deep belly) fat, Tesamorelin is especially useful for women who carry weight around their organs. It mimics growth hormone–releasing hormone (GHRH), promoting fat loss while preserving lean tissue.

Combining Lifestyle with Peptides

Peptides work best when paired with smart choices. You do not need extreme dieting or punishing workouts, but you do need alignment. Focus on:

- A high-protein, moderate-carb, low-sugar diet
- Strength training 2–3 times per week
- Stress management and good sleep hygiene
- Intermittent fasting if appropriate

When your body is no longer in survival mode, fat becomes fuel again.

Most women notice better sleep, reduced bloating, and improved energy within 2–3 weeks. Visible fat loss typically begins around week 4–6. With consistent use, belly fat begins to shrink, waistlines tighten, and inflammation subsides.

Don't be mistaken. Peptides do not force your body into weight loss. ***They remove the roadblocks, so your body can do what it's meant to do***: thrive, burn, and balance.

If you've tried everything and nothing works, this might be your missing piece. Belly fat is not your fault. But with the right tools, it no longer has to be your struggle.

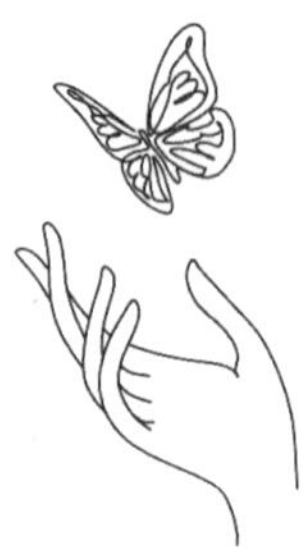

Semaglutide, Tirzepatide, and Appetite Control

For women dealing with weight gain, especially around midlife, controlling appetite is half the battle. Even with clean eating and regular movement, constant hunger, cravings, or emotional eating can sabotage progress. This is where GLP-1 receptor agonists like Semaglutide and Tirzepatide have changed the game.

Originally developed for type 2 diabetes, these peptides have shown powerful benefits in regulating appetite, promoting satiety, and supporting sustainable fat loss.

Unlike stimulant-based suppressants, they work with the body's hormonal cues, which makes them highly effective and surprisingly well-tolerated.

How Semaglutide and Tirzepatide Work

Semaglutide mimics GLP-1 (glucagon-like peptide-1)—a hormone released in the gut when you eat. GLP-1 tells your brain that you're full, slows stomach emptying, and reduces food cravings.

This leads to smaller portions, fewer snacks, and more control over hunger signals.

Together, these peptides help reset your relationship with food—not by force, but by enhancing natural fullness cues that have dulled over time due to stress, hormone shifts, or overeating.

Benefits Beyond Appetite Control

- Steady, consistent fat loss
- Lower insulin and blood sugar levels
- Improved portion control without hunger
- Increased confidence and body awareness
- Reduced risk of weight regain

Many women describe a calmness around food that they haven't felt in years. It becomes easier to say no, easier to stop at one serving, and easier to enjoy food without guilt.

Weight loss tends to be steady, averaging 1 to 3 pounds per week, with noticeable reductions in waist size by month two. The best part is that it feels natural. You eat less because you're actually full, not because you're pushing through cravings.

How They're Taken

Both Semaglutide and Tirzepatide are injectable, taken subcutaneously once per week. Doses are titrated slowly to avoid nausea or digestive side effects. These peptides are now widely available through telehealth services and should be administered under medical guidance.

Combining with Other Peptides

To maximize results, some women stack Semaglutide or Tirzepatide with:

- CJC-1295 + Ipamorelin (for metabolism and recovery)
- BPC-157 (for gut health)
- AOD-9604 (for targeted fat breakdown)

For women tired of dieting drama, these peptides offer clarity, balance, and finally—results. ***Hunger no longer controls your day. You do.***

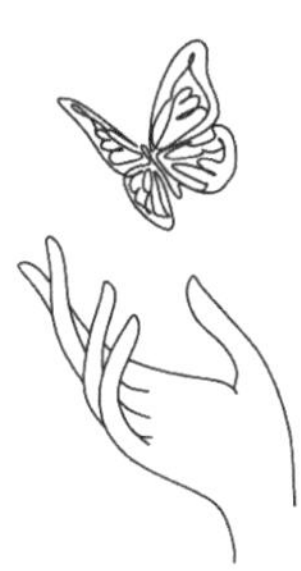

Growth Hormone Secretagogues

As women enter their late 30s and 40s, growth hormone levels naturally decline. This decrease may not be immediately obvious, but its effects are felt everywhere—from slower metabolism and increased body fat to decreased muscle tone, dull skin, and longer recovery times. For women seeking to optimize aging and body composition, ***growth hormone secretagogues like CJC-1295 and Ipamorelin*** offer a powerful and targeted solution.

Unlike synthetic human growth hormone (HGH) injections, which can disrupt the body's own hormone rhythms, secretagogues gently stimulate the ***pituitary gland to release your body's natural HGH***, preserving balance while still delivering transformative benefits.

What Are Growth Hormone Secretagogues?

Secretagogues are peptides that encourage your own body to release growth hormone in controlled pulses, mimicking the way it worked when you were younger.

Among them, two of the most widely used are:

- **CJC-1295 (with DAC)**: Mimics growth hormone–releasing hormone (GHRH), promoting a long-lasting increase in HGH levels.
- **Ipamorelin**: A growth hormone–releasing peptide (GHRP) that stimulates the pituitary without affecting cortisol or prolactin. It has a clean safety profile and is well tolerated.

When combined, these peptides work to elevate and prolong the natural secretion of growth hormone, leading to enhanced recovery, fat burning, and cellular repair, and all without any side effects.

Benefits for Women

- Fat Loss: Especially around the abdomen, hips, and thighs—areas where stubborn fat accumulates with age.
- Muscle Preservation and Growth: Ideal for women engaging in strength training or trying to prevent age-related muscle loss (sarcopenia).
- Improved Sleep: Deeper, more restorative sleep, which boosts metabolism and energy.
- Better Recovery: From workouts, injury, or general stress.
- Enhanced Mood and Focus: Thanks to better sleep and hormonal balance.

How They Are Used

CJC-1295 and Ipamorelin are typically administered together via subcutaneous injection once daily, usually at night to mimic the body's natural growth hormone pulse during sleep. Dosing is customized, but most protocols last 12 to 16 weeks, with a break before restarting to prevent tolerance.

This nightly injection stimulates a slow and steady rise in HGH over weeks—offering a safer, more natural alternative to direct HGH therapy.

Who Is It For?

- Women over 40 looking to improve energy and body composition
- Perimenopausal and postmenopausal women experiencing fatigue, weight gain, and decreased muscle tone
- Anyone wanting to age with vitality, preserve lean mass, and avoid hormonal imbalances

Because growth hormone plays a role in almost every system—from metabolism to cell repair—its gentle stimulation helps the entire body work more efficiently.

Unlike stimulants or diet pills, results are ***gradual but lasting***. Most women notice better sleep, improved skin tone, and more energy within 2–4 weeks. Fat loss, especially in the midsection, becomes noticeable around week 6–8. Muscle tone and recovery improvements follow soon after.

CJC-1295 and Ipamorelin represent a smart, safe, and sustainable way to ***turn back the biological clock*** by reminding the body how to function like before.

For women seeking to feel stronger, look leaner, and age gracefully, ***growth hormone secretagogues are one of the most promising tools in modern peptide therapy***. Gentle, effective, and deeply rejuvenating, they offer a new path to lasting health and beauty.

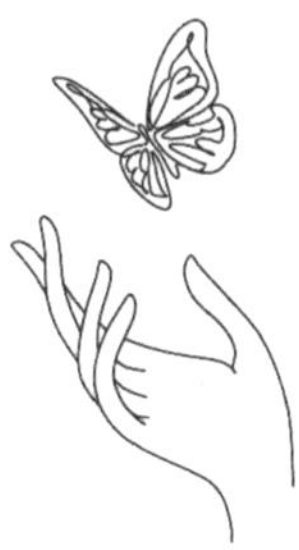

Body Sculpting and Muscle Toning over 40

Many women over 40 face a frustrating reality: no matter how well they eat or how often they exercise, their body no longer responds the way it once did. Muscle mass decreases. Fat deposits settle in stubborn areas. And the definition they once had seems harder to regain.

This is not a failure of effort. It is the biology of aging. After 35, women lose about 1% of muscle mass per year. Hormonal shifts—especially the decline of estrogen and growth hormone—slow down metabolism and make it easier to store fat. But with the right approach, ***it is entirely possible to sculpt a lean, strong, toned physique well into your 40s, 50s, and beyond.***

Peptides are a powerful addition to this strategy.

They do not replace exercise or nutrition—but they make both work better by restoring the signals that support lean tissue, metabolism, and recovery.

Why Muscle Matters More After 40

Muscle is not just about aesthetics. It is your metabolic engine. More muscle means:

- Higher resting metabolism
- Better insulin sensitivity
- Stronger bones
- Improved mobility and posture
- Greater hormonal balance

As women age, preserving and building muscle becomes less about "looking fit" and more about health, longevity, and confidence.

Peptides That Support Body Sculpting

- **CJC-1295 + Ipamorelin**: Stimulates growth hormone release, supporting fat metabolism and lean muscle development. Recovery improves, workouts feel more productive, and body composition shifts more easily.
- **AOD-9604**: Targets fat-burning pathways without affecting muscle mass. Great for reducing adipose tissue in the belly and thighs.
- **Tesamorelin**: Shown to reduce visceral fat, which is especially important for cardiovascular and metabolic health.

- **BPC-157 and TB-500**: Help with recovery from workouts, joint inflammation, and connective tissue repair. This allows women to train more consistently without injury setbacks.
- **5-Amino-1MQ**: A newer peptide that enhances muscle endurance and energy production by increasing NAD+ and improving cellular metabolism.

Training + Peptide = Results

Peptides do not build muscle on their own. They enhance the results of training, especially resistance or strength training.

Ideally, your weekly routine should include:

- 3 strength training sessions (bodyweight, bands, or weights)
- 1–2 mobility or functional movement sessions (yoga, pilates, stretching)
- Daily movement (walking, light cardio)
- Recovery days with sleep, hydration, and proper nutrition

When this is paired with a peptide protocol that supports hormonal and metabolic health, body recomposition becomes truly realistic.

Body sculpting after 40 is not out of reach. It simply requires smarter strategies that align with your evolving biology. Peptides provide the support your body craves to build strength, burn fat, and recover faster.

This is not a quick fix. It is a long-term upgrade. When you combine intelligent movement with cellular-level support, you get results that are not only visible—but sustainable. ***Strong is not a phase. It is your foundation for everything that comes next.***

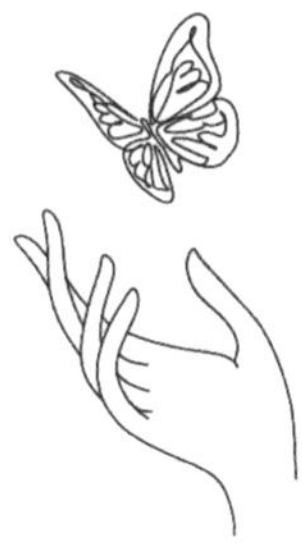

Part IV:
Peptides for Vitality, Libido, and Energy

Sexual Wellness with Peptides

For many women, changes in sexual desire are deeply personal and often difficult to talk about. As hormones shift with age, childbirth, stress, or menopause, libido can begin to fade—sometimes subtly, sometimes drastically. This is not about a lack of love or attraction. It is about biology. And thankfully, ***biology can be supported.***

Peptides offer a new, effective, and science-backed path to restoring ***female sexual desire, arousal, and pleasure*** without hormonal chaos or side effects. They work with the body to enhance the systems that naturally spark intimacy, making them one of the most exciting advancements in modern sexual wellness.

Unlike men, female libido is more complex, involving physical, emotional, and neurological signals. This is why peptide therapy can be so powerful. It supports multiple layers of this experience.

Why Libido Declines for Women

There are many reasons why a woman may experience a drop in sexual desire:

- Hormonal changes (decline in estrogen, testosterone, oxytocin)
- Stress and cortisol overload
- Fatigue or poor sleep
- Vaginal dryness or reduced blood flow
- Psychological factors: anxiety, body image, past trauma

Unlike hormone replacement therapy, these peptides do not flood your system with synthetic hormones. Instead, they support natural responses, making them safer and more adaptable to your needs.

When to Use Libido Peptides

These peptides can be used:

- As-needed before intimacy (like PT-141)
- In a short cycle to rebalance hormones (like Kisspeptin)
- Ongoing in small doses for mood and connection (like Oxytocin)

They can also be stacked with energy or mood peptides for an even more complete wellness approach.

Top Libido-Enhancing Peptides for Women

- ***PT-141 (Bremelanotide)***: This peptide is specifically approved for treating low sexual desire in women. It works in the brain, activating receptors tied to arousal and motivation—not just genital blood flow. It helps women feel mentally and physically in the mood. PT-141 is taken via injection or nasal spray and usually takes effect within a few hours.
- ***Kisspeptin-10***: A reproductive peptide that stimulates luteinizing hormone and can help rebalance sexual hormones like testosterone and estrogen. Useful for women in perimenopause or those experiencing low libido due to hormonal imbalances.
- ***Oxytocin*** (the "bonding hormone"): Often compounded as a nasal spray, oxytocin enhances emotional closeness, pleasure sensitivity, and post-orgasm bonding. It helps improve mood and intimacy in long-term relationships.

Peptides are powerful, but they work best in harmony with lifestyle support, like healthy fat intake, sleep, exercise, and stress reduction.

Sexual wellness is not just about pleasure. It is about confidence, connection, and vitality. You deserve to feel alive in every area of your life.

With the right peptide support, ***libido is not something you have to mourn.*** It is something you can reignite. Your body still remembers how to respond. It just needs the right signal.

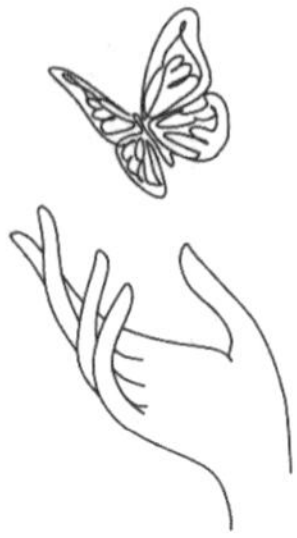

Sleep, Recovery, and the Power of Sermorelin

Sleep is the foundation of wellness, especially as we age.

Yet, for many women over 35, sleep becomes lighter, more fragmented, and less restorative. You might wake up at 3 a.m. and struggle to fall back asleep. You may sleep eight hours but still feel drained. If this sounds familiar, your growth hormone levels may be declining—and with them, your body's ability to repair, burn fat, and recharge fully.

Enter *Sermorelin*, a peptide that gently stimulates the body's natural growth hormone production, helping you not only sleep deeper, but recover stronger.

Why Growth Hormone and Sleep Are Connected

Growth hormone is primarily released during deep sleep, especially in the early phases of the night. It supports tissue repair, fat metabolism, cognitive function, and even emotional resilience.

As women age and enter perimenopause or menopause, ***growth hormone production declines***—often alongside changes in estrogen and progesterone. This decline disrupts sleep architecture. You spend less time in deep, restorative stages, and more time in light, unrefreshing cycles. As a result:

- Recovery slows
- Fatigue builds
- Mood suffers
- Muscle tone fades
- Brain fog becomes common

By restoring the natural rhythm of growth hormone, Sermorelin helps rebuild this essential connection between sleep and repair.

What Is Sermorelin?

Sermorelin is a growth hormone–releasing hormone (GHRH) analog, meaning it mimics the body's natural signals to trigger growth hormone production from the pituitary gland. ***It is not synthetic HGH.*** Instead, it works by encouraging your body to release its own hormones—making it safer and more physiologically aligned.

Benefits of Sermorelin for Women

- Deeper, uninterrupted sleep
- Faster physical recovery from workouts or stress
- Improved skin quality and hydration
- Fat loss (especially visceral fat)
- Enhanced cognitive function and mood stability
- Greater muscle tone and bone strength

Many women describe waking up refreshed, clear-headed, and energized for the first time in years.

To amplify its effects:

- Maintain a regular sleep schedule
- Avoid blue light and screens before bed
- Include strength training and protein-rich meals
- Limit sugar and alcohol, which suppress growth hormone

It is especially effective for those who are not ready for hormone replacement therapy but want a gentle, regenerative boost.

You can also pair Sermorelin with CJC-1295 + Ipamorelin for a deeper peptide stack that targets immediate and extended growth hormone release.

Sleep is not just rest. It is when your body rebuilds. *If you are not sleeping well, you are not healing.*

Sermorelin helps correct that at the hormonal root. It is not a sedative. It is not a stimulant. It is a biological reset switch, guiding your body back into its natural rhythm—so that each night becomes a time of true renewal.

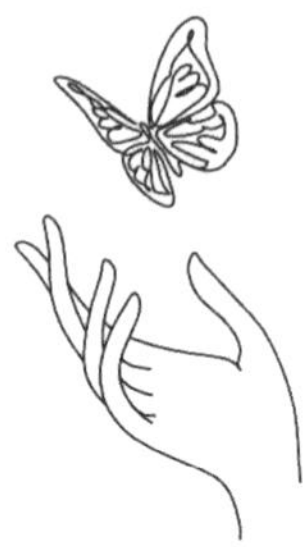

Increasing Energy, Focus, and Cognitive Function

Mental clarity and lasting energy are two of the first things women notice slipping away with age. Tasks that were once simple feel draining. Words hang just out of reach. Focus fractures.

Many women chalk it up to stress or being busy, but the truth often lies deeper. Declines in estrogen, growth hormone, thyroid function, and mitochondrial health all play a role. Fortunately, peptide therapy offers real solutions to help restore your cognitive edge and sustain your energy throughout the day.

Your brain thrives on clear communication between neurons, strong blood flow, and stable neurotransmitter levels. When these systems falter, you feel it. Fatigue sets in. Brain fog clouds your mornings. Even your creativity and memory can dull.

Peptides help reset your system, giving you back the ability to think clearly and live purposefully.

Key Peptides for Mental Energy and Focus

1

Selank
A neuropeptide that *promotes focus, reduces anxiety, and improves memory retention.* Selank increases serotonin and dopamine activity in the brain, which helps regulate attention and mood. It is often used by people who want sharper thinking without the jittery side effects of stimulants.

2

Semax
This peptide is known for its *cognitive-enhancing effects.* It works by increasing levels of brain-derived neurotrophic factor (BDNF), which helps form new neural connections. Semax is especially helpful during periods of burnout or brain fatigue.

3

MOTS-c
A mitochondrial peptide that *enhances cellular energy production.* By supporting your mitochondria, MOTS-c helps increase overall stamina and reduces the sense of physical and mental exhaustion. It also improves glucose metabolism and metabolic efficiency.

4

CJC-1295 + Ipamorelin
Though often used for *fat loss and muscle tone*, these peptides also improve *sleep quality and recovery*, which in turn helps you wake up more energized and alert.

Benefits You Can Expect

- Increased mental sharpness
- More stable energy throughout the day
- Faster recovery from stress or cognitive overload

These peptides are most effective when taken consistently. Some come in nasal spray form, others via subcutaneous injection.

Supporting Brain Health Holistically

While peptides provide powerful support, it is important to pair them with habits that protect cognitive health:

- Get 7 to 9 hours of quality sleep
- Eat omega-3 rich foods like fish, walnuts, and flaxseed, and reduce sugar and processed carbs\
- Move your body daily, even with gentle exercise
- Take breaks from screens to reduce mental fatigue

Peptides help you get back in control. Not just of your body. But of your mind.

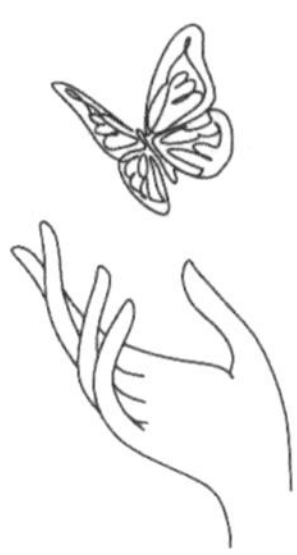

Mood, Motivation, and Menopause Relief

Mood swings. Sudden tears. Irritability over the smallest things. Feeling numb or emotionally distant.

For many women, these are the symptoms of hormonal shifts that begin in perimenopause and intensify through menopause. Estrogen, progesterone, and testosterone all play a role in emotional regulation. As they decline, so does your resilience.

But that does not mean you have to live with it. Peptides offer a gentle and effective way to support your mood, motivation, and emotional well-being during this stage of life.

Menopause affects the brain just as much as the body. Lower estrogen levels can reduce serotonin and dopamine production, leading to anxiety, depression, and even a loss of drive or joy. Peptides can help restore that balance by improving neurotransmitter activity and supporting the hormonal systems that influence your emotions.

Peptides for Mood and Menopause Balance

- **Selank**: Known for its anti-anxiety and mood-stabilizing effects, Selank helps improve emotional resilience without sedation. It increases levels of GABA and serotonin, creating a calm and steady emotional baseline.
- **Oxytocin**: Often called the "love hormone," oxytocin fosters connection, reduces stress, and enhances feelings of closeness and warmth. It can be especially helpful for women navigating changes in intimacy during menopause.
- **Kisspeptin**-10: This peptide influences reproductive hormones and may help re-stimulate natural hormone production in the early stages of perimenopause. It has shown promise in boosting mood and motivation by balancing estrogen and testosterone.
- **Tesamorelin or CJC-1295 + Ipamorelin**: These peptides promote deep sleep and energy recovery, indirectly helping stabilize mood. Better rest often translates into fewer emotional fluctuations.
- **Thymosin Alpha-1**: This immune-modulating peptide also plays a role in reducing inflammation, which is closely linked to mood disorders. It supports overall vitality and reduces the emotional drain from chronic stress.

Your body is adapting to a new hormonal rhythm. With the right support, you do not have to suffer through it.

Peptides offer that support. They help bring back lightness. Joy. Drive. And peace.
Menopause is not the end of vitality. It can be the beginning of a more powerful, more balanced version of you.

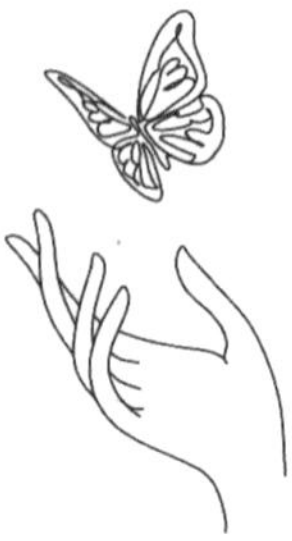

Part V: Protocols, Stacks, and Personalized Plans

Choosing the Right Peptides for Your Goals

The world of peptides is exciting, but for many women, it can also feel overwhelming. With dozens of peptides available—each promising something different—it's easy to get lost in the options. One targets fat loss. Another improves sleep. A third regenerates skin. So where do you begin?

The answer depends entirely on your personal goals.

Peptides are tools, not magic pills. The right one will align with your unique needs, current health status, and the specific outcomes you're hoping to achieve.

Choosing well means understanding how each peptide works, and how it fits into your overall wellness journey.

This chapter will help you take the guesswork out of peptide selection and give you the clarity and confidence to get started.

Step 1:
Get Clear on Your Priorities

Start by identifying your top three wellness goals. These are the changes that would most impact your day-to-day life. Examples might include:

- Losing body fat (especially around the belly)
- Getting deeper, more restorative sleep
- Rebuilding muscle tone and energy
- Restoring libido and intimacy
- Improving skin elasticity and glow
- Reducing inflammation or joint pain
- Managing mood or brain fog during menopause

Once you're clear on what matters most, the peptide landscape becomes much easier to navigate.

Step 2:
Match Your Goal to the Peptide

Use the table to find peptide matches for your goals.

Goal	**Recommended Peptides**	**Primary Effects**
Fat loss	CJC-1295 + Ipamorelin, AOD-9604, Tesamorelin	Increases metabolism, reduces visceral fat
Sleep & recovery	Sermorelin, CJC-1295, Epitalon	Improves deep sleep, boosts growth hormone

Goal	Recommended Peptides	Primary Effects
Muscle tone & strength	Ipamorelin, 5-Amino-1MQ, MOTS-c	Supports endurance, cellular energy
Skin rejuvenation	GHK-Cu, Matrixyl, SNAP-8	Smooths wrinkles
Hair regrowth	GHK-Cu, BPC-157, TB-500	Enhances follicle health
Libido & sexual wellness	PT-141, Oxytocin, Kisspeptin-10	Increases desire and emotional connection
Mood & cognition	Selank, Semax, Thymosin Alpha-1	Reduces anxiety, boosts mental clarity
Menopause support	Kisspeptin-10, CJC-1295, Oxytocin	Balances hormones

These peptides are often used in combination, called "stacks," to address multiple goals at once.

Step 3:
Understand Your Hormonal Landscape

Age, menstrual status, stress, sleep, and overall health all impact your hormonal profile. A woman in early perimenopause may need very different support than a postmenopausal woman dealing with long-term inflammation and fatigue.

You do not always need bloodwork before starting peptide therapy, but it can help. Basic panels like hormone levels (estradiol, progesterone, testosterone), thyroid, insulin, and cortisol offer insight into what your body may need most. A telehealth practitioner or functional medicine specialist can help interpret results and suggest the most appropriate peptide approach.

Step 4:
Consider Delivery Method and Lifestyle Fit

Some peptides require daily or weekly injections. Others come as nasal sprays or topical serums. If you are new to biohacking, starting with a topical peptide like GHK-Cu for skin or a nasal spray like Selank for focus may be an easy entry point.

On the other hand, if you are committed to major transformation—like fat loss or muscle toning—injectables such as CJC-1295 or Tesamorelin will offer the most powerful results.

Your comfort level matters.

Think about your routine. Are you likely to remember a daily protocol? Would a once-a-week injection be easier? Your lifestyle can shape your success, so choose a protocol that fits seamlessly into your day.

Step 5: Monitor, Cycle, and Adjust

Peptides are not a one-size-fits-all solution. Results often build over weeks, and subtle shifts—like better sleep or reduced cravings—are sometimes the first signs it's working. Track your progress with:

- Photos every 2–4 weeks
- A wellness journal for mood, energy, sleep, libido, etc.
- Simple body measurements (waist, thighs, hips)
- Monthly check-ins with a practitioner if possible

After 8–12 weeks, most peptides are cycled off to prevent tolerance. You can then rotate to a different peptide or take a short break before restarting.

Choosing the right peptides begins with choosing yourself. Your goals. Your body. Your future. Whether you want to tone up, think sharper, feel sexier, or age with grace, there is a protocol that can help.

Peptides are not a shortcut, but they are support. And with the right match, they become one of the most powerful tools you can use to step into your next chapter with energy, clarity, and confidence. You deserve nothing less.

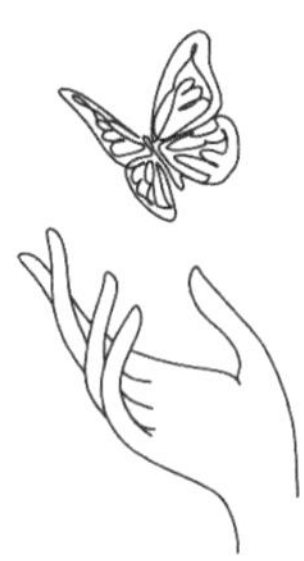

Stacking: What Works Best Together

Peptide stacking is the art of combining multiple peptides to enhance results. Think of it like a well-balanced skincare routine or a workout plan that targets strength, flexibility, and endurance all at once. When done correctly, stacking amplifies benefits while keeping your protocols efficient and aligned with your goals.

What Is Stacking?

Stacking = Synergy
Using 2–3 peptides together that complement each other for a stronger, more holistic effect. The goal is not to overload but to target multiple systems at once—fat loss, energy, sleep, skin, libido—based on your unique goals.

Here's a simple, visually organized guide to help you stack like a pro.

Stack 1:

Beauty + Anti-Aging Glow

Peptide	Function
GHK-Cu	Boosts collagen, skin repair, hair regrowth
Matrixyl	Smooths wrinkles, improves skin elasticity
SNAP-8	Softens expression lines, firms skin

How to use:

Apply topically as part of your morning and evening skincare routine. Microneedle weekly for enhanced results.

Stack 2:

Fat Loss + Body Sculpting

Peptide	Function
CJC-1295 + Ipamorelin	Boosts HGH, fat burning, and lean muscle
AOD-9604	Targets stubborn fat without affecting muscle
MOTS-c	Increases energy and metabolism at the cellular level

How to use:

Inject subcutaneously 1x daily
(usually at night) for 8–12 weeks.
Combine with strength training for best results.

Stack 3:

Libido + Hormonal Support

Peptide	Function
PT-141	Increases sexual desire and arousal
Oxytocin	Enhances connection, intimacy, and pleasure
Kisspeptin -10	Balances reproductive hormones naturally

How to use:

PT-141 can be taken as needed.
Oxytocin and Kisspeptin work best in short cycles.
Always consult your provider.

Stack 4:

Mental Clarity + Mood Boost

Peptide	Function
Selank	Reduces anxiety, improves focus
Semax	Increases BDNF for cognitive health

How to use:

Nasal spray (Selank/Semax) daily in the morning. Thymosin Alpha-1 by injection 2–3 times weekly.

General Tips for Stacking

✓ Limit to 2–3 peptides per cycle to keep things simple and trackable

✓ Cycle off every 8–12 weeks to avoid resistance and give your body time to reset

✓ Stay hydrated, eat clean, and prioritize sleep to amplify your results

✓ Track your progress using a journal or weekly check-ins

Conclusion

The power of peptides lies in personalization. Stacking allows you to tailor your protocol to exactly what your body needs.

Start small. Stay consistent.

And let your body show you just how good it can feel.

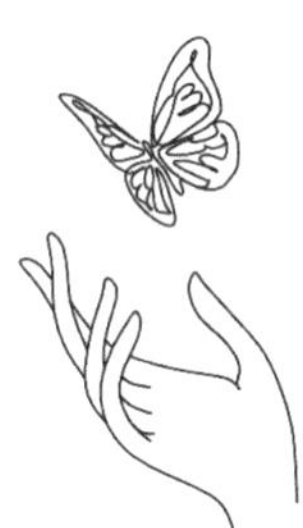

Injection Guide, Cycling Plans, and Side Effect Management

If you're new to peptides, the idea of giving yourself injections may feel intimidating.

But the truth is, subcutaneous injections are simple, safe, and nearly painless when done correctly.

This step-by-step process will explain how to cycle peptides effectively, and help you stay aware of possible side effects and how to manage them.

Injection Guide: How to Inject Peptides Safely
Peptides used for fat loss, muscle growth, sleep, and recovery are most often administered subcutaneously—just beneath the skin into the fatty layer, typically around the abdomen or thigh.

What You'll Need:

- Insulin syringes (29–31 gauge, 0.5 or 1 mL)
- Alcohol wipes
- Your reconstituted peptide vial
- A sterile vial of bacteriostatic water (for mixing)
- A sharps container for disposal

Step-by-Step Process:

1. **Wash your hands thoroughly** with soap and water.
2. **Wipe the peptide vial** and the bacteriostatic water vial with alcohol.
3. **Draw up water** into the syringe and slowly inject it into the peptide vial (usually 1–2 mL depending on protocol).
4. **Gently swirl** (don't shake) the vial to mix. Store it in the refrigerator.
5. To inject, **draw the appropriate dose into the syringe**. Tap to release air bubbles.
6. **Choose an injection site** (abdomen or upper thigh). Wipe it clean with an alcohol pad.
7. **Pinch the skin** and insert the needle at a 45–90° angle. Inject slowly.
8. **Dispose of the needle** safely in a sharps container.

With practice, this becomes a quick and easy part of your routine, often taking less than 2 minutes per day.

Cycling Plans: How Long to Use Peptides

To keep peptides effective and avoid receptor fatigue, most are used in *cycles of 8 to 12 weeks*, followed by a 2 *to 4 week break*.

Sample Cycles:

- ***CJC-1295 + Ipamorelin***: 8–12 weeks on, 4 weeks off
- ***GHK-Cu (topical)***: Continuous use is fine
- ***PT-141***: Taken as needed or in short bursts
- ***Semaglutide/Tirzepatide***: Can be used longer term under supervision
- ***Selank/Semax***: 10–14 days on, 7 days off

Why cycle?

Cycling gives your body time to reset and maintain sensitivity to the peptide. It also allows you to assess progress and avoid dependency or plateau.

During your "off" period, you can continue supportive habits like clean eating, strength training, hydration, and sleep tracking.

You may also switch to different peptides for new goals.

Side Effect Management: What to Watch For

While peptides are generally well tolerated, mild side effects may occur—especially during the first 1–2 weeks as your body adjusts.

Common Mild Side Effects:

- Redness or itching at injection site
- Mild bloating or water retention
- Temporary fatigue or headache
- Nausea (especially with Semaglutide or PT-141)
- Hunger or mood changes (linked to hormonal shifts)

These are usually temporary and fade with continued use or slight dose adjustments.

Less Common Reactions:

- Insomnia (from dosing peptides too late in the day)
- Dizziness or light-headedness (from rapid hormonal shifts)
- Injection site bruising (use a new site each day)

Tips to Reduce Side Effects:

- Always start with the lowest effective dose
- Take peptides at consistent times, ideally morning or evening depending on type
- Stay hydrated to flush excess byproducts
- Rotate injection sites to reduce irritation
- Use professional-grade peptides from trusted sources only

Peptides are powerful, but they work best when used ***intelligently, consistently, and safely***. Mastering injections, understanding cycles, and knowing how to respond to side effects gives you full control of your transformation journey.

This is not about perfection. It is about ***empowered experimentation***. With the right guidance and self-awareness, you can use peptides as long-term allies in your health, beauty, and vitality. Let your body do what it was designed to do—heal, strengthen, and shine.

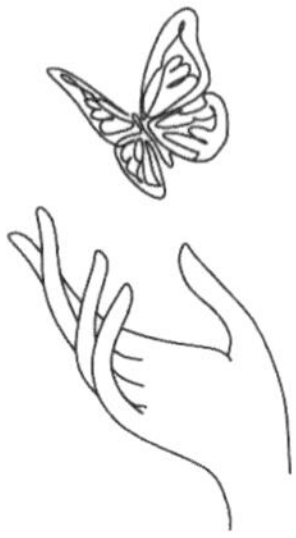

Part VI: Transformation Programs

14-Day Peptide Jumpstart Program

If you are just starting your peptide journey, a 14-day protocol is the perfect way to ease in, observe changes, and build momentum. While peptides work best over time, the first two weeks often bring powerful shifts—better sleep, reduced cravings, increased mental clarity, and subtle changes in skin texture or mood. This short plan is designed to gently activate your body's natural repair systems without overwhelm.

Program Goals

- Prime your body for fat loss and muscle recovery
- Improve sleep and mental energy
- Begin skin repair and hydration
- Reduce inflammation and increase daily vitality

You will focus on three core peptide goals:
Sleep + Recovery,
Fat Metabolism, and
Skin & Mood Boost

Peptides Used in This Protocol

Peptide	Purpose	Dosage/Timing
CJC-1295 + Ipamorelin	Stimulates HGH for fat loss and sleep	Inject 1x daily at night before bed
GHK-Cu (topical)	Enhances collagen, improves skin tone	Apply serum morning and night to face/neck
Selank (nasal spray)	Reduces anxiety, increases focus	1–2 sprays per nostril in the morning

Morning

- Apply GHK-Cu serum after cleansing
- Use Selank nasal spray
- Hydrate with warm lemon water and take omega-3s or multivitamin
- Eat a protein-rich breakfast (eggs, protein smoothie, Greek yogurt)

Midday

- Walk or light exercise (15–30 mins)
- Stay hydrated and avoid processed sugar

Evening

- Eat dinner 3 hours before bed (light protein + veggies)
- Inject CJC-1295 + Ipamorelin 30 minutes before sleep
- Journal mood, energy, cravings, and skin observations
- Power down screens 60 minutes before bed

Weekly Goals

Week 1

- Sleep quality improves
- Cravings begin to lessen
- Slight skin glow appears
- Better mood and focus in mornings

Week 2

- Less bloating and inflammation
- Deeper, more restorative sleep
- More energy throughout the day
- Improved hydration and skin tone
- Subtle fat loss around midsection for some

Pro Tips for Success

✓ Stay consistent with timing. Hormones respond to rhythm.
✓ Don't skip hydration. Peptides are more effective when the body is well hydrated.
✓ Limit sugar and alcohol. These disrupt hormonal signals and reduce peptide efficiency.
✓ Move your body, even gently, with walks, stretching, or light resistance training.

What to Expect After 30 Days

You may not see a dramatic physical transformation just yet, but you will likely feel more **rested, calmer, sharper, and energized**. Your skin may look smoother, and your waistline may start to feel less inflamed.

Most importantly, you'll have built the foundation for deeper transformation ahead. The 14-day program is your reset button. If you're ready, the next phase—30 days—will take your results to the next level.

In the next section, we'll guide you through building on this base with more targeted stacks and protocols for fat loss, strength, and glow.

30-Day Peptide Transformation Plan

Once you've completed your 14-day peptide jumpstart, your body is primed. You've likely started noticing better sleep, a calmer mood, and subtle changes in your skin or energy. The 30-day transformation builds on that foundation to target body composition, mental sharpness, libido, and skin health in a more focused and visible way.

Goals for the 30-Day Plan

- Accelerate fat burning and muscle toning
- Deepen sleep and support natural growth hormone pulses
- Improve mood, motivation, and mental clarity
- Stimulate collagen and tighten the skin
- Gently enhance libido and energy

Build Momentum.
Sculpt Your Body.
Recharge Your System.

Peptides Used in This Protocol

Peptide	Purpose	Dosage/Timing
CJC-1295 + Ipamorelin	Boost HGH for fat loss, muscle tone, sleep	Inject once nightly
GHK-Cu (topical)	Stimulates collagen, smooths fine lines	Apply serum twice daily
PT-141 (optional)	Enhances sexual desire and arousal	Use as needed (2x weekly max)

Morning

- Selank spray (1–2 sprays per nostril)
- Inject AOD-9604 before food
- Apply GHK-Cu serum after cleansing
- Protein-rich breakfast (scrambled eggs, avocado, or a smoothie)

Afternoon

- Light physical activity (walking or strength workout)
- Hydrate and eat whole foods
- Track how your body feels (energy, mood, hunger)

Evening

- Apply GHK-Cu serum again
- Inject CJC-1295 + Ipamorelin 30 minutes before bed
- PT-141 as needed (optional and based on libido support days)
- No screens 1 hour before sleep, and lights out before 10:30 p.m.

Weekly Focus Areas

Week 1

- Recalibrate your energy and sleep rhythms
- Curb cravings and reduce bloating
- Feel clearer and calmer in the mornings

Week 2

- Skin begins looking brighter and smoother
- Deeper sleep, fewer nighttime wakeups
- Subtle waistline tightening, especially with AOD-9604

Week 3

- More defined body shape and stamina
- Mood becomes more stable and uplifted
- Libido boost for those using PT-141

Week 4

- Slimmer midsection, glowing skin
- Enhanced self-confidence and body awareness
- Better connection with routines

Tips for Maximum Results

✓ Avoid alcohol and sugar, which disrupt peptide signaling
✓ Prioritize sleep—7 to 9 hours is key
✓ Stay hydrated, aiming for 2 to 3 liters daily
✓ Stack with resistance training 2–3x per week for body recomposition
✓ Use a journal to track sleep, mood, weight, skin, and libido progress

Expected Outcomes After 30 Days

- Noticeable fat loss in stubborn areas
- Healthier skin tone and texture
- Sharper focus and more balanced moods
- Improved sleep and morning energy
- A renewed sense of motivation and wellness

This 30-day plan is your reset and reawakening. Your body is responding. Your mind is clearer. You're not just looking better—you're feeling alive again. Up next, the 60-day plan takes your progress and turns it into a long-term lifestyle. ***Let's keep going.***

What to Expect After 60 Days

You may not see a dramatic physical transformation just yet, but you will likely feel more **rested, calmer, sharper, and energized**. Your skin may look smoother, and your waistline may start to feel less inflamed.

Most importantly, you'll have built the foundation for deeper transformation ahead. The 14-day program is your reset button. If you're ready, the next phase—30 days—will take your results to the next level.

In the next section, we'll guide you through building on this base with more targeted stacks and protocols for fat loss, strength, and glow.

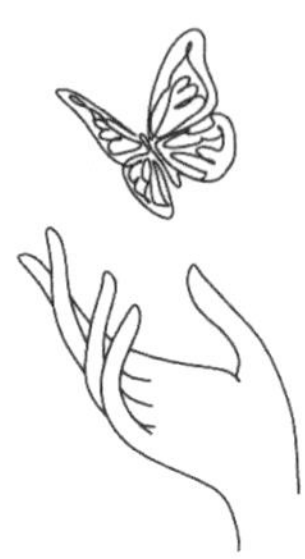

60-Day Peptide Transformation Plan

If you've completed the 30-day peptide program, you've already experienced clearer skin, better sleep, renewed energy, and visible fat loss. Now, with the next 30 days, the goal is lasting change. This phase is about locking in results and pushing your transformation further—on the inside and out.

Goals for Days 31–60

- Accelerate fat loss and muscle tone
- Support hormonal balance through perimenopause or menopause
- Continue skin rejuvenation and reduce fine lines
- Optimize brain function, mood, and clarity
- Boost endurance, energy, and recovery capacity
- Establish sustainable wellness routines

Deep Body recomposition.
Lasting beauty.
Full-System renewal.

Peptides Used in This Protocol

Peptide	Purpose	Dosage/Timing
CJC-1295 + Ipamorelin	Deepens fat burning, recovery, and muscle tone	Inject once nightly before bed
GHK-Cu (topical)	Smooths skin, tightens texture, supports hair	Apply twice daily
MOTS-c	Boosts cellular energy, metabolic resilience	Inject 2–3x per week (morning)
PT-141 or Oxytocin	Enhances libido and intimacy	Use 1–2x weekly as needed
Selank or Semax	Maintains focus, reduces stress and anxiety	Daily nasal spray (morning)
AOD-9604	Continues fat breakdown	Inject in the morning daily

Morning

- MOTS-c and AOD-9604 injection
- Selank or Semax spray
- Apply GHK-Cu serum
- Hydrating breakfast: protein + healthy fats + fiber

Afternoon

- Movement session: weight training, Pilates, or walking
- Balanced lunch with lean protein, greens, and complex carbs
- Stay hydrated and mindful of stress

Evening

- Second application of GHK-Cu serum
- Inject CJC-1295 + Ipamorelin 30 minutes before sleep
- PT-141 or Oxytocin (on planned evenings for libido support)
- Lights out routine: no screens, calming music or journaling

Weekly Focus Map

Week 5

- Fat loss continues noticeably
- Muscles feel firmer and workouts more effective
- Skin looks lifted and more hydrated

Week 6

- Mood feels more stable, stress responses soften
- Libido support feels more natural and consistent
- Waistline shrinks, posture improves, energy is steady

Week 7

- More defined abs, arms, and facial contour
- Brain fog is rare—focus sharpens
- Skin glows even without makeup

Week 8

- Wellness becomes routine
- Body feels light, strong, and confident
- Strong sleep cycles and emotional clarity

Maximize This Phase

✓ **Keep stacking smart:** Don't add more than 3–4 peptides total

✓ **Sleep is sacred:** Hormonal regeneration needs full rest

✓ **Protein is your best friend:** 80–120g per day for muscle support

✓ **Track progress weekly:** Photos, journaling, mood logs, waist measurement

✓ **Hydrate like it's your job:** Skin, fat loss, and mitochondria rely on it

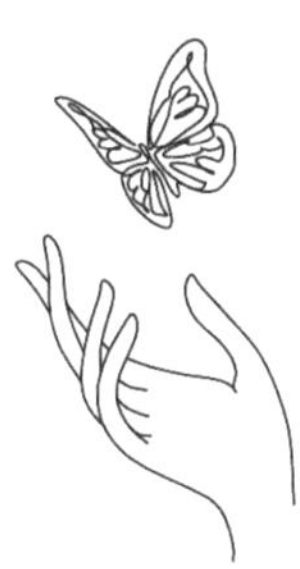

What You Can Expect After 60 Days

- A visibly leaner, sculpted physique
- Firmer skin, brighter eyes, reduced inflammation
- Stronger libido and emotional connection
- Faster recovery from stress and workouts
- Enhanced confidence and mental clarity
- A new baseline of energy and vitality

You've now completed a full-body reset—not through restriction or extremes, but through targeted cellular support. You're not only aging well, **you're rewriting what aging looks like.**

The next step? Sustain the glow. Cycle smart. Stack for your seasons. And know that the transformation is no longer temporary. It's your new normal.

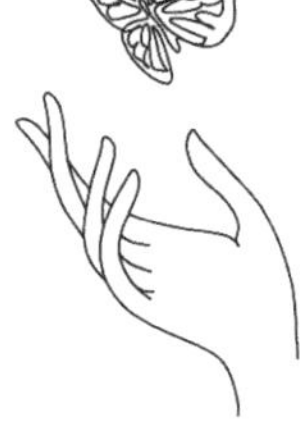

Part VII: Long-Term Wellness and Advanced Biohacking

Anti-Aging and Mitochondrial Health

Aging is often seen as a slow surrender: a gradual breakdown of skin, energy, memory, and strength. But what if aging was not simply a matter of time, but of biology? What if the key to living longer and looking younger lies not in your birthdate, but in your mitochondria?

This chapter focuses on the science of cellular aging, the role of mitochondrial health, and how peptides can support longevity and vibrancy from the inside out. It is not just about staying alive longer. It is about feeling strong, capable, and radiant in every season of life.

Why Mitochondria Matter in Aging

Mitochondria are often called the "powerhouses of the cell." They create ATP, the energy your cells use to function. Everything from brain activity to skin repair to fat metabolism depends on mitochondrial output.

Live stronger, longer,
and brighter from the inside out.

As you age, mitochondria weaken and multiply more slowly. Damaged mitochondria produce less energy and more oxidative stress. This leads to:

- Chronic fatigue
- Brain fog
- Muscle loss
- Wrinkling and sagging skin
- Slower metabolism
- Inflammatory disorders

In other words, mitochondrial decline is a core driver of aging. To slow aging, you need to restore mitochondrial function. And peptides can help.

Visible and Invisible Benefits

While the benefits of mitochondrial peptides often begin at the cellular level, they become visible in powerful ways:

- Increased daily energy without caffeine
- Reduced inflammation and joint stiffness
- Clearer skin, stronger hair, and brighter eyes
- Improved sleep and hormonal rhythm
- Mental sharpness and mood stability
- Slower signs of physical aging

Peptides like MOTS-c and Epitalon often make people feel “lit from within”—an alert, light, focused sensation that builds over time.

Peptides That Support Mitochondrial Health

1

MOTS-c
A mitochondrial-derived peptide that enhances glucose metabolism, improves insulin sensitivity, and boosts cellular resilience. MOTS-c helps the body adapt to stress and burns energy more efficiently, making it ideal for fat loss and anti-aging. It is typically injected 2–3 times per week.

2

5-Amino-1MQ
A peptide that blocks the NNMT enzyme, which slows metabolism in aging cells. It encourages fat cells to burn more energy and helps prevent mitochondrial decline. This peptide is associated with improved endurance, fat loss, and cognitive energy.

3

Epitalon
A pineal gland–derived peptide known to lengthen telomeres, which are protective caps on the ends of DNA strands. Longer telomeres are associated with longer life and reduced risk of age-related disease. Epitalon also improves melatonin production and deep sleep.

4

BPC-157
Though best known for healing injuries, BPC-157 also reduces oxidative stress and inflammation—two major causes of cellular aging.

These peptides are not cosmetic fixes. They restore energy at the source, protecting your cells from decay and dysfunction.

Supporting Longevity Beyond Peptides

Peptides are tools, but the foundation of anti-aging remains lifestyle-based. Combine your protocol with:

- ***Deep sleep***: This is when mitochondria repair and regenerate
- ***Exercise***: Especially resistance training and zone 2 cardio
- ***Nourishing food***: Colorful vegetables, healthy fats, and clean protein
- ***Stress control***: Chronic cortisol damages mitochondrial DNA
- ***Cold exposure or sauna***: Encourages cellular resilience and detox

Use peptides as accelerators, not replacements. Let them amplify the efforts you're already making.

The Big Picture

Longevity is not about denying age. It is about thriving in it. When your cells are healthy, your whole body performs better. You move with energy. Think with clarity. Feel youthful not just in appearance, but in how you live your life.

Peptides for mitochondrial health help slow the clock from the inside. They restore vitality, reverse fatigue, and allow your body to regenerate at the cellular level.

Aging is not a countdown. It is a choice to show up stronger, smarter, and brighter—with every passing year. Let your mitochondria lead the way.

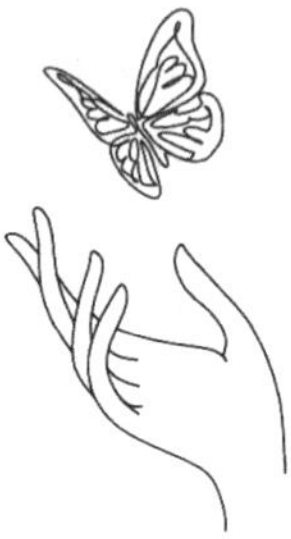

Peptides, Regenerative Medicine, and Cellular Rejuvenation

Regenerative medicine is the frontier of modern healing. Instead of suppressing symptoms, it focuses on helping the body repair, restore, and regenerate itself. At the center of this revolutionary approach are peptides—tiny but powerful molecules that speak the body's natural language of renewal.

From smoother skin and stronger joints to faster injury recovery and reduced inflammation, ***peptides offer a targeted way to activate your body's built-in repair systems***. This is not about quick fixes or superficial results. This is about changing the way your body heals and thrives at the cellular level.

Heal at the Root, not the Surface.

What Is Regenerative Medicine?

Regenerative medicine aims to rebuild damaged tissues, revive cell function, and reverse degenerative processes. It's used in everything from orthopedics and aesthetics to gut repair and chronic fatigue treatment.

At its heart, regenerative medicine believes that your body doesn't need to be forced to heal—it needs to be reminded. Peptides do just that.

They bind to receptors on cells and send signals that trigger regeneration, growth, and anti-inflammatory processes.

How Peptides Help You Regenerate

Unlike pharmaceuticals that often override systems, peptides are highly selective. They target specific repair mechanisms based on your body's current needs. Some support collagen synthesis, others heal tissue injuries, while some reduce inflammation in the gut, brain, or joints.

Here are four key regenerative peptides every woman should know.

Peptides That Support Mitochondrial Health

1

BPC-157 (Body Protection Compound)
Stimulates angiogenesis (formation of new blood vessels)
Repairs gut lining, tendons, ligaments, and muscles
Excellent for women with gut issues, workout injuries, or chronic inflammation
Typically injected subcutaneously near the site of pain or taken orally for gut repair

2

TB-500 (Thymosin Beta-4)
Promotes cell migration and tissue remodeling
Enhances wound healing and reduces scar tissue
Useful for joint pain, tendon injuries, or post-surgical recovery
Often stacked with BPC-157 for full-body repair support

3

GHK-Cu (Copper Peptide)
Accelerates skin regeneration, tightens loose skin
Heals small wounds, reduces scarring, and promotes hair growth
Applied topically or injected for facial rejuvenation and anti-aging

4

Thymosin Alpha-1
Regulates immune response and reduces chronic inflammation
Ideal for women with autoimmune conditions, chronic fatigue, or post-viral symptoms
Works systemically to balance the immune system and support long-term healing

Tissue Repair vs. True Rejuvenation

Most treatments reduce pain or inflammation temporarily.

Peptides change the structure and function of cells over time, allowing the body to regenerate stronger, healthier tissue.

For example:

- A sprained knee can recover faster and stronger with TB-500 and BPC-157
- A leaky gut can heal with BPC-157, improving digestion, nutrient absorption, and mood
- Postpartum skin laxity or hair thinning can be reversed with GHK-Cu
- Low immunity and chronic fatigue can improve with Thymosin Alpha-1

This is **true rejuvenation**. It's rebuilding, not masking.

When and How to Use Regenerative Peptides

- Post-injury or surgery: Speeds healing and reduces downtime
- During intense training: Prevents overuse injuries

- In chronic inflammation: Restores tissue health and reduces autoimmune flare-ups
- As part of an anti-aging routine: Supports muscle, joint, skin, and organ health

Most are used subcutaneously, either systemically (like Thymosin Alpha-1) or locally (like BPC-157 near an injury). Stacking multiple peptides is often recommended, depending on the issue.

Your body was built to heal. Peptides help it remember how. Let peptides lead the repair from within.

Regenerative peptides are about capability.
About moving without pain.
Thinking without fog. Aging without decay.

Supporting Skin, Hormones, and Metabolism Naturally

Beautiful skin, balanced hormones, and a fast, efficient metabolism are not just surface goals—they're signs of inner balance. For women, especially over 35, these three systems become deeply interconnected. When one shifts, the others follow. If your skin is dull, your hormones may be fluctuating. If your metabolism has slowed, inflammation or hormonal resistance may be the cause. The good news? You can support all three systems naturally—using peptides, habits, and targeted nutrition that help your body reset from the inside out.

This chapter focuses on how to ***nourish your skin, regulate your hormones, and boost metabolism*** with peptide therapy and simple wellness strategies that truly work.

Whole-body harmony, without overwhelm.

1. Glowing, Resilient Skin from Within

Your skin reflects what's happening inside your body. Starting in your late 20s, collagen production declines by about 1% per year. By 40, you may notice increased dryness, fine lines, and sagging. Instead of layering on more creams, stimulate your skin to repair itself.

Key Peptides for Skin:

- **GHK-Cu**: Increases collagen and elastin production, fades discoloration, improves firmness
- **Matrixyl**: Targets wrinkles and boosts skin density
- **SNAP-8**: Softens expression lines and improves smoothness

How to use: Apply topically twice daily. Use microneedling 1x weekly to enhance absorption. Support your routine with hydration and sleep.

Peptides work better when your skin is not inflamed. Avoid harsh exfoliants and prioritize gentle, nourishing routines. A calm, well-fed skin barrier holds moisture and repairs faster.

2. Hormonal Balance Without Chaos

Women's hormones shift every month, and more dramatically during perimenopause and menopause. When estrogen, progesterone, and testosterone dip or fluctuate, symptoms like hot flashes and mood swings appear.

Rather than replacing hormones with aggressive therapies, peptides help gently stimulate natural balance.

Key Peptides for Hormonal Support:

- ***Kisspeptin-10***: Encourages the release of reproductive hormones
- ***PT-141***: Boosts sexual desire and arousal by acting on the brain, not just hormones
- ***Thymosin Alpha-1***: Calms autoimmunity and chronic inflammation that interfere with hormone signaling
- ***CJC-1295 + Ipamorelin***: Supports healthy growth hormone rhythm, improving sleep and hormone regulation

How to use: Injections are done daily or weekly depending on the peptide. Work with a provider to adjust doses.

3. Reigniting a Sluggish Metabolism

As estrogen drops, so does metabolic rate. The result? Fat gain, especially around the belly, along with fatigue and reduced stamina. Peptides can help by restoring mitochondrial efficiency, reducing insulin resistance, and supporting lean muscle development.

Key Peptides for Metabolism:

- *AOD-9604*: Promotes fat breakdown and reduces adipose tissue
- *MOTS-c*: Boosts cellular energy and glucose utilization
- *5-Amino-1MQ*: Enhances metabolism at the cellular level and helps with body recomposition

How to use: Inject daily or 2–3x per week depending on the peptide.

Lifestyle habits matter here, too. Prioritize protein, magnesium, and B vitamins. Reduce caffeine and alcohol which disrupt hormone balance. Other natural supports include time-restricted eating, prioritizing sleep, and managing stress.

The Natural Alignment of All Three

You do not need to chase separate solutions for every symptom. ***When your skin, hormones, and metabolism are aligned, everything improves together.*** Your glow returns. Your energy is steady. Your body feels like home again.

Start simple. Pick one peptide stack that supports two of these systems. Adjust slowly. Stay consistent. Your body will respond, not because you forced it—but because you supported it.

This is not about perfection. It is about balance. And when your inner systems are nourished naturally, your outer results become inevitable.

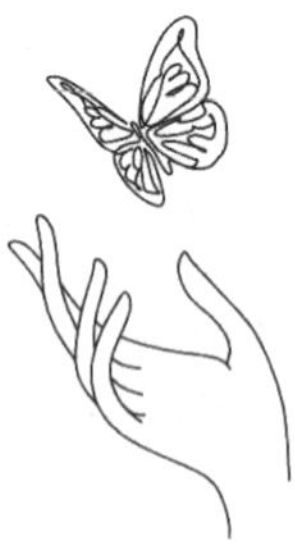

Creating a Sustainable Beauty and Wellness Routine

True beauty and wellness do not come from short-term detoxes, endless product swaps, or unrealistic routines. They come from sustainable systems—***the small, consistent actions you take each day*** that nourish your body, support your hormones, and build lasting confidence.

Here we focus on how to create a balanced, realistic wellness routine using peptides, rituals, and lifestyle habits that align with your long-term goals.

Whether you want to keep glowing skin, a sculpted body, balanced mood, or lasting energy, the secret lies in designing a plan you enjoy sticking to.

1. Build Your Foundation First

A sustainable beauty and wellness routine starts with foundational habits, not fancy extras. Think of it as your daily checklist that supports cellular repair, hormonal balance, and mental clarity.

The Core Four

✓ ***Hydration***: Aim for at least 2–3 liters of water daily

✓ ***Protein***: Eat 80–120g of protein daily to support skin, muscle, and hormones

✓ ***Sleep***: Prioritize 7–9 hours of deep, uninterrupted sleep

✓ ***Movement***: Include daily walking and strength training 2–3x a week

Peptides work best when your body is already getting the basics. These habits amplify results and make every drop of effort count.

2. Choose Peptides That Fit Your Life

You don't need every peptide. Choose 2–3 that align with your main goals. This keeps your routine simple and reduces burnout or decision fatigue.

Example of Sustainable Stacks:

- ***CJC-1295 + Ipamorelin***: For sleep, fat loss, and muscle tone
- GHK-Cu (topical): For skin tightening and glow
- ***Selank***: For mood, focus, and emotional balance

Set your peptides up with reminders or place them next to your toothbrush, skincare products, or water bottle. ***The easier it is to remember, the more likely you'll stay consistent.***

3. Stack Habits for Better Consistency

Attach new habits to existing ones. For example:

- Use peptide nasal spray right after brushing your teeth
- Apply your serum after setting your morning coffee
- Do a 5-minute stretch while your skincare soaks in

Habit stacking turns routines into second nature. Soon, your wellness rituals feel like just another part of you.

4. Create Daily Beauty Rituals

Instead of rushing through your skincare routine, make it a daily moment of self-connection. This boosts emotional wellness, lowers stress, and makes consistency feel more joyful than rigid.

Morning Ritual

- Cleanse gently
- Apply GHK-Cu serum and hyaluronic acid
- Use Selank nasal spray if needed
- Take a moment to breathe or speak a positive affirmation

Evening Ritual

- Cleanse, apply peptides and moisturizer
- Inject CJC-1295 + Ipamorelin 30 minutes before bed
- Power down electronics, sip tea, or stretch
- Reflect in a journal or plan your next day with intention

5. Embrace a Flexible Mindset

Sustainability does not mean perfection. Life will bring travel, off-days, emotional dips, and skipped workouts. ***Instead of quitting or starting over, shift your mindset to flexibility.***

Missed a dose?
Continue tomorrow.
Traveled without your peptides?
Focus on water and sleep.
Ate off-plan? Nourish better at the next meal.

Progress is not linear. What matters most is the long-term rhythm, not the occasional misstep.

6. Track, Reflect, Adjust

Every 30 days, check in with yourself:
How is your sleep, skin, energy, and mood?
Do you feel supported by your current stack?
What's feeling easy? What's feeling hard?

Make adjustments slowly.
Let your wellness evolve with your life.

A sustainable beauty and wellness routine is about support, not stress. It works with your body, not against it. ***With the right peptides, daily rituals, and habits you actually enjoy, you can look and feel better for years to come.***

This is not about 'chasing youth'. You're owning your vitality with grace and ease. Your beauty is not something to fix. It's something to nourish—day by day, breath by breath. And now, you have everything you need to do just that.

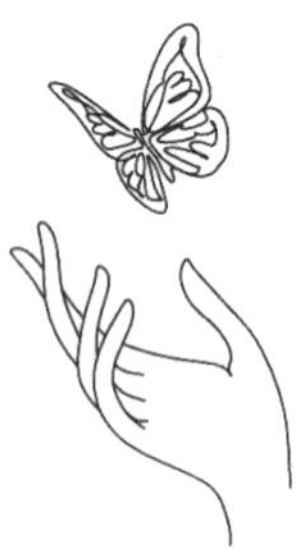

Conclusion & References

Rewriting the Narrative

For far too long, women have been told that aging is something to fight, hide, or fear. We are surrounded by messages that imply youth is the only time we're allowed to feel beautiful, energetic, or desirable. But that story is outdated. It is time to rewrite the narrative—because the truth is, you can look and feel younger, stronger, and more vibrant at any stage of life.

You can look and feel younger.

Aging is not a decline. It is a transition—a shift in your biology that, with the right support, can be just as powerful as any other phase. You are not losing yourself. You are meeting a new version of you—one who is wiser, more resilient, and still capable of glowing from the inside out.

You do not have to accept fatigue, weight gain, brain fog, or dry skin as your new normal. You do not have to disappear into the background as the years go by.

Your best days are not behind you. They are ahead of you—if you choose to support your body with care, science, and intention.

True confidence does not come from looking perfect. It comes from feeling in tune with your body. It's in the way you walk into a room with energy. It's in the glow of rested skin, the lift in your voice, the strength in your steps. And it comes from knowing that you are taking care of yourself—not just for how you look, but for how you live.

Peptides are tools, not trophies. They help you nurture what's already within—your vitality, your radiance, your power. When used consistently and mindfully, they restore balance, reduce inflammation, and reawaken parts of you that felt dimmed by time or stress. This is beauty from within, regenerated, not disguised.

Ageless living is not about denying age. It is about embracing every chapter with more energy, more clarity, and more freedom. ***It is knowing that glowing skin, lean strength, and deep connection are available at any age, not just in your 20s.***

You deserve to feel vibrant. You deserve to feel sexy, centered, and strong—without apology or limitation.

So take this knowledge. Build your rhythm. Choose the routines that nourish you deeply. Let peptides support the incredible machine that is your body. And ***walk forward with grace***, not in fear of aging, but in celebration of the life still unfolding.

This is your time. You are not behind. You are right on time. And your next chapter will be your strongest yet.

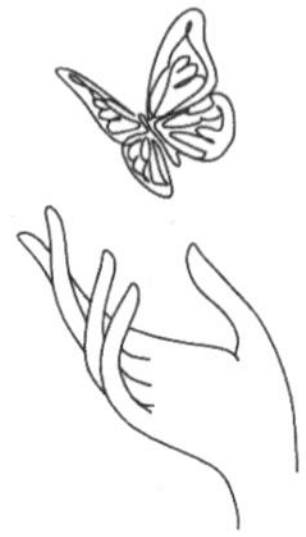

Where to Buy Trusted Peptides

With the growing popularity of peptides, the market is filled with options—but not all are safe, legal, or effective. Choosing a trusted source is one of the most important decisions you'll make on your peptide journey. ***The quality, purity, and legitimacy of your peptides directly impact your results and safety.***

This section will help you understand what to look for in a supplier and where to buy peptides with confidence.

Why Quality Matters

Peptides are delicate compounds. They must be properly synthesized, handled, and stored to maintain their stability and potency. If you buy from an unverified source, you risk receiving:

- Impure or contaminated product
- Incorrectly dosed formulas
- Bacterial exposure
- Peptides that degrade before reaching your body

Even worse, some black-market peptides are diluted with unknown fillers or mislabeled entirely. These products may not just be ineffective—they could be dangerous.

Trusted Sources: What to Look For

1

U.S.-Based or Internationally Regulated Pharmacies
Choose compounding pharmacies or telehealth clinics licensed to dispense medical-grade peptides. These typically require a consultation or prescription, which adds an extra layer of protection.

2

Customer Support and Reviews
Look for websites with real reviews, transparent contact options, and clear return/refund policies. Avoid sellers that hide behind anonymous web pages or push "research only" disclaimers without explanation.

3

Cold Chain Shipping
Some peptides, like CJC-1295 or Ipamorelin, are temperature-sensitive. Vendors should ship with cold packs or clearly state how products are preserved.

4

Certificate of Analysis (CoA)
Reputable sellers provide third-party lab reports showing purity, sterility, and concentration of their peptides. If no CoA is offered, that's a red flag.

5

Medical Oversight or Telehealth Access
Some trusted sources now offer online consultations with providers who can recommend personalized protocols and ship peptides to homes.

Top Options for Buying Trusted Peptides

While specific vendor names can change over time, here are the types of sources to seek out:

- ***Licensed Compounding Pharmacies***: Offer the highest-grade injectable peptides under physician supervision
- ***Telehealth Platforms*** (U.S. based): Provide consults, prescriptions, and pharmacy fulfillment
- ***Functional Medicine Clinics***: Often dispense topical and injectable peptides directly to patients
- ***Specialty Peptide Distributors***: Some trusted companies offer over-the-counter cosmetic peptides like GHK-Cu for topical use

Be cautious of vendors that label products "for research purposes only" but market them for human use. This is a legal loophole and not a reliable source for personal health products.

Peptides are powerful. ***They work best when they're clean, dosed properly, and stored correctly.*** Investing in high-quality products from licensed sources is not just safer—it gives you peace of mind that what you're using is real, active, and supportive of your transformation.

When in doubt, work with a licensed provider or certified functional medicine practitioner to guide your purchases and protocol. With the right source and support, your peptide journey can be safe, effective, and deeply rewarding.

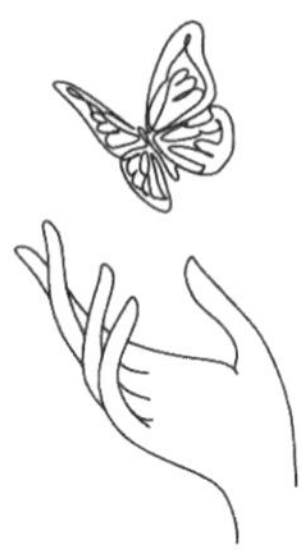

Tools

Peptides by Purpose: A Summary

Fat Loss & Body Composition

- **CJC-1295 + Ipamorelin** – Stimulates growth hormone for fat burning and recovery
- **AOD-9604** – Targets adipose tissue, especially stubborn belly fat
- **Tesamorelin** – Reduces visceral fat
- **5-Amino-1MQ** – Enhances metabolism and cellular energy
- **MOTS-c** – Improves mitochondrial function and fat oxidation

Skin, Hair & Beauty

- **GHK-Cu (Copper Peptide)** – Boosts collagen, reduces wrinkles, improves skin tone
- **Matrixyl** – Targets wrinkles and increases skin density
- **SNAP-8** – Relaxes facial tension lines
- **PTD-DBM + Valproic Acid** – Activates hair follicle regeneration
- **TB-500 + BPC-157** – Promote hair regrowth and skin healing

Hormonal & Sexual Health

- **PT-141 (Bremelanotide)** – Enhances libido and sexual arousal
- **Kisspeptin-10** – Regulates reproductive hormones
- **Oxytocin** – Boosts intimacy, bonding, and mood
- **Thymosin Alpha-1** – Reduces inflammation and balances immunity

Energy, Mood & Focus

- **Selank** – Improves anxiety, focus, and memory
- **Semax** – Enhances cognitive performance and resilience
- **MOTS-c** – Increases endurance and energy
- **5-Amino-1MQ** – Supports cognitive clarity via NAD+ and energy metabolism

Recovery, Sleep & Repair

- **Sermorelin** – Improves sleep and recovery by boosting natural HGH
- **Epitalon** – Regulates melatonin, supports deep sleep, and extends telomere health
- **CJC-1295 + Ipamorelin** – Improves deep sleep and body repair

Peptide Stacks by Goal

Goal	Stack
Skin + Glow	GHK-Cu + Matrixyl + SNAP-8 (topical)
Fat Loss + Metabolism	CJC-1295 + Ipamorelin + AOD-9604 + MOTS-c
Libido + Hormonal	PT-141 + Oxytocin + Kisspeptin-10
Focus + Energy	Selank + Semax + MOTS-c
Recovery + Sleep	Sermorelin + Epitalon + BPC-157

Tools & Resources

Injection Supplies

- Insulin syringes (29–31 gauge, 0.5–1 mL)
- Alcohol wipes
- Bacteriostatic water for reconstitution
- Sharps disposal container

Application Aids

- Microneedling device (0.5 mm for skin penetration)
- Derma rollers for scalp or skin
- Storage: Cool packs or refrigeration for temperature-sensitive peptides

Tracking Tools

- Daily peptide log or habit tracker
- Wellness journal: for sleep, energy, mood, and libido
- Progress photos and weekly measurements

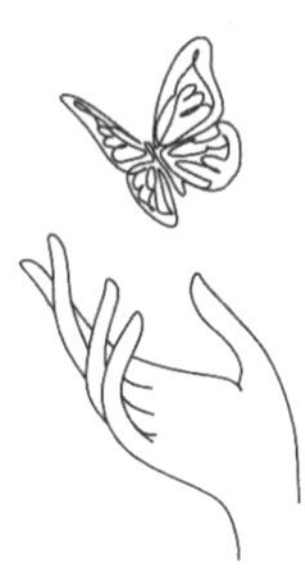

PEPTIDE TRACKER

Name:
Energy Levels: _____/10
Mood: _____/10
Notes:

Date	Time	Peptides taken & site	Dose

WEEKLY REFLECTION

(Use this journal to keep track of your transformation programs)

Best improvement noticed this week:

Any side effects or discomforts?

Next week's goals or changes:

WEEKLY REFLECTION

(Use this journal to keep track of your transformation programs)

Best improvement noticed this week:

Any side effects or discomforts?

Next week's goals or changes:

WEEKLY REFLECTION

(Use this journal to keep track of your transformation programs)

Best improvement noticed this week:

Any side effects or discomforts?

Next week's goals or changes:

WEEKLY REFLECTION

(Use this journal to keep track of your transformation programs)

Best improvement noticed this week:

____

____

____

____

____

____

Any side effects or discomforts?

____

____

____

____

____

____

Next week's goals or changes:

____

____

____

____

____

____

WEEKLY REFLECTION

(Use this journal to keep track of your transformation programs)

Best improvement noticed this week:

Any side effects or discomforts?

Next week's goals or changes:

WEEKLY REFLECTION

(Use this journal to keep track of your transformation programs)

Best improvement noticed this week:

____

____

____

____

____

____

Any side effects or discomforts?

____

____

____

____

____

____

Next week's goals or changes:

____

____

____

____

____

____

WEEKLY REFLECTION

(Use this journal to keep track of your transformation programs)

Best improvement noticed this week:

Any side effects or discomforts?

Next week's goals or changes:

WEEKLY REFLECTION

(Use this journal to keep track of your transformation programs)

Best improvement noticed this week:

Any side effects or discomforts?

Next week's goals or changes:

WEEKLY HABITS TRACKER

(Use this tracker to track your transformation programs)

List of Activities	Mon	Tue	Wed	Thu	Fri	Sat	Sun
Drink water after waking							
Resistance training							
Eat healthy breakfast							
Take a walk outside							
Limited sugar & alcohol							
Protein for muscle							
Sleep							

SELF-REFLECTION NOTE:

WEEKLY HABITS TRACKER

(Use this tracker to track your transformation programs)

List of Activities	Mon	Tue	Wed	Thu	Fri	Sat	Sun
Drink water after waking							
Resistance training							
Eat healthy breakfast							
Take a walk outside							
Limited sugar & alcohol							
Protein for muscle							
Sleep							

SELF-REFLECTION NOTE:

WEEKLY HABITS TRACKER

(Use this tracker to track your transformation programs)

List of Activities	Mon	Tue	Wed	Thu	Fri	Sat	Sun
Drink water after waking							
Resistance training							
Eat healthy breakfast							
Take a walk outside							
Limited sugar & alcohol							
Protein for muscle							
Sleep							

SELF-REFLECTION NOTE:

WEEKLY HABITS TRACKER

(Use this tracker to track your transformation programs)

List of Activities	Mon	Tue	Wed	Thu	Fri	Sat	Sun
Drink water after waking							
Resistance training							
Eat healthy breakfast							
Take a walk outside							
Limited sugar & alcohol							
Protein for muscle							
Sleep							

SELF-REFLECTION NOTE:

WEEKLY HABITS TRACKER

(Use this tracker to track your transformation programs)

List of Activities	Mon	Tue	Wed	Thu	Fri	Sat	Sun
Drink water after waking							
Resistance training							
Eat healthy breakfast							
Take a walk outside							
Limited sugar & alcohol							
Protein for muscle							
Sleep							

SELF-REFLECTION NOTE:

WEEKLY HABITS TRACKER

(Use this tracker to track your transformation programs)

List of Activities	Mon	Tue	Wed	Thu	Fri	Sat	Sun
Drink water after waking							
Resistance training							
Eat healthy breakfast							
Take a walk outside							
Limited sugar & alcohol							
Protein for muscle							
Sleep							

SELF-REFLECTION NOTE:

WEEKLY HABITS TRACKER

(Use this tracker to track your transformation programs)

List of Activities	Mon	Tue	Wed	Thu	Fri	Sat	Sun
Drink water after waking							
Resistance training							
Eat healthy breakfast							
Take a walk outside							
Limited sugar & alcohol							
Protein for muscle							
Sleep							

SELF-REFLECTION NOTE:

WEEKLY HABITS TRACKER

(Use this tracker to track your transformation programs)

List of Activities	Mon	Tue	Wed	Thu	Fri	Sat	Sun
Drink water after waking							
Resistance training							
Eat healthy breakfast							
Take a walk outside							
Limited sugar & alcohol							
Protein for muscle							
Sleep							

SELF-REFLECTION NOTE:

WEIGHT LOSS TRACKER

MONTH: YEAR:

DATE	WEIGHT	GAIN+	LOSS+	NOTES

WORKOUT JOURNAL

Date ________________

Time/distance ________________

Notes ________________

____

____

Rate your workout ○○○○○

Date ________________

Time/distance ________________

Notes ________________

____

____

Rate your workout ○○○○○

Date ________________

Time/distance ________________

Notes ________________

____

____

Rate your workout ○○○○○

Date ________________

Time/distance ________________

Notes ________________

____

____

Rate your workout ○○○○○

Date ________________

Time/distance ________________

Notes ________________

____

____

Rate your workout ○○○○○

Date ________________

Time/distance ________________

Notes ________________

____

____

Rate your workout ○○○○○

FOOD JOURNAL

Breakfast

Monday
Tuesday
Wednesday
Thursday
Friday
Saturday
Sunday

Rate your week ○○○○○

Lunch

Monday
Tuesday
Wednesday
Thursday
Friday
Saturday
Sunday

Rate your week ○○○○○

Dinner

Monday
Tuesday
Wednesday
Thursday
Friday
Saturday
Sunday

Rate your week ○○○○○

Snacks

Monday
Tuesday
Wednesday
Thursday
Friday
Saturday
Sunday

Rate your week ○○○○○

Notes:

WELLNESS TRACKER

NAME ____________________ **DATE** ____________________

Key/Day	1	2	3	4	5	6	7	8	10	9	11	12	13	14	15	16	17	18	19	20	21	22	23	24	25	26	27	28	29	30
Stress Level																														
Mood Rating																														
Mental Clarity																														
Happiness																														
Gratitude																														
Counseling																														
Relaxation																														
Hobbies																														
Screen Time																														
Journaling																														

Notes

To Do Next